Strength Training
for the over
50s

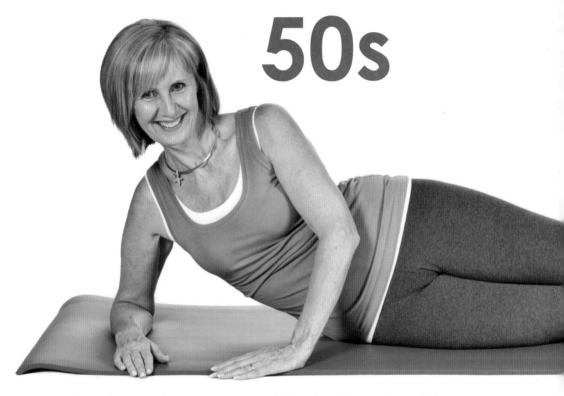

Staying strong and healthy for life

John Forde

The Five Mile Press

The Five Mile Press Pty Ltd
1 Centre Road, Scoresby
Victoria 3179 Australia
www.fivemile.com.au

First published 2010

Printed in China

Cover and page design by Aimee Zumis
Photography by Peter Bourne
Illustrations by Gaston Vanzet
Images pp123-125 courtesy of Shutterstock

National Library of Australia Cataloguing-in-Publication entry
    Author: Forde, John.
    Title: Strength training for the over 50s : staying strong and healthy for life / John Forde.

    ISBN: 9781742480473 (hbk.)

    Subjects: Exercise for middle aged persons.
    Physical fitness for middle aged persons.
    Exercise for older people.
    Physical fitness for older people.

    Dewey Number: 613.0434

Contents

About the Models

About the Models

Liz Simpson is 58 years old and last year learned to do the splits for the first time. She has been involved with artistic rollerskating for almost 30 years, and is currently involved in coaching and choreographing the routines for The Pacemakers, the only team of adult rollerskaters in Australia. For almost 11 years Liz has also had a great interest in tai chi, and is currently working towards her black sash. Under the tuition of her Masters, she has discovered that you are never too old to learn or to get stronger, fitter and more flexible. Be it in skating, tai chi or life in general, Liz is a firm believer in the 3P's … Practice, Perseverance and Patience. Oh yes, and plenty of chocolate!

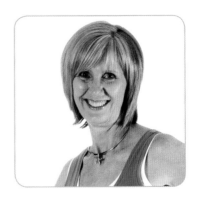

Terry Lees is an active 55-year-old, and the father of three great kids, now pretty much grown up. He is a geologist with a career in mineral exploration which has taken him to many out-of-the-way places in Australia and overseas – travelling has always been part of his life. Terry keeps fit and healthy through exercise and a good diet, and believes in the motto 'Use it or lose it'. He practices taekwondo and is training for his black-belt grading. He also swims regularly, rides to work and goes to the gym. Terry is based in Melbourne with his lovely partner Dianne.

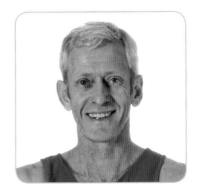

Joan Green is 61 years old, married with two adult children, and runs an interior design business. Joan has always been active, playing tennis and squash when younger and, more recently, skating in an adult precision routine. Joan is a yoga devotee, enjoys ballroom and Latin dancing, and firmly believes in regular exercise and strength work.

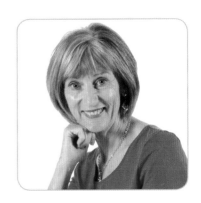

Chapter 1 Introduction

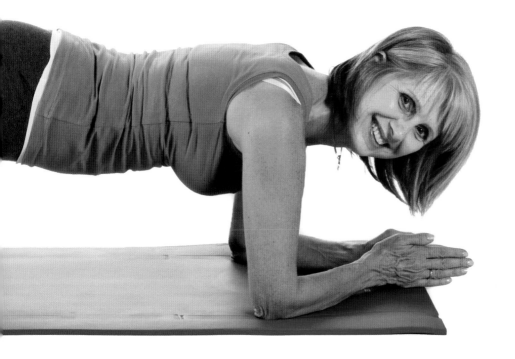

The Importance of Strength Training for Older Adults

As life goes on, we age. This is the one thing of which we can all be sure. The good thing is that, as individuals, we do have control over the quality of life we live while on this earth. It is possible to reverse the ageing process. For too long, many people have believed that as we age we must inevitably get weaker, suffer more aches and pains, lose muscle and gain fat. But the truth is that most of these conditions are caused by an unhealthy lifestyle, including years of inactivity.

In actual fact, with a little change of their routine, everyone has the potential to live a fulfilling life in their older years. You do not need to give in to inactivity, declining abilities and infirmity. Every year medical advances are ensuring longer life expectancies, enabling people to live lives that extend far beyond that of our ancestors. This is causing us to reassess the way we look after ourselves.

All over the world, doctors and fitness experts are recommending strength training for patients to help prevent age-related deterioration in muscle, bone density and metabolism. As well, strength training is beneficial in reducing risk of injury, increasing strength and helping with weight management. Furthermore, research suggests strength training also helps treat, better manage and prevent back pain, arthritic discomfort, diabetes, osteoporosis and high blood pressure.

To assist in preventing and minimising age-related health problems and conditions it is important we keep active. Being active helps maintain ongoing independence so we can take care of ourselves. Strength training will improve our strength and bone density, and attending stretches and balance training will help to ensure we maintain a good range of movement.

An increase in strength can help with your everyday life making it easier and more enjoyable, whether you are carrying your shopping, attending to your gardening, enjoying recreational activities or walking the dog. Furthermore, the more you exercise, the easier it will become. You will notice your endurance levels improve as well.

Now that we know how good strength training is for us, let's talk about what strength training is. Strength training is described as briefly working your muscles on a regular basis beyond what they are accustomed to. This causes the muscles to become stronger and larger. Your tendons, ligaments and bones will also strengthen, causing your joints to become more stable, which in turn will lower your risk of injury.

Would you like to stay fit, trim, strong and mobile well into your older years? If so, then don't accept frailty and the various limitations of age. Do something about it. Even if you suffer from a medical condition, strength training can help reduce the risk of developing other conditions, and improve your current medical condition.

How Much Physical Activity Should I Be Doing?

It is recommended that every healthy person undertakes a good variety of regular physical activity. On a daily basis, take every opportunity you can to be active without exhausting yourself and eventually this will become habit. Walk to the shops rather than drive. Take the stairs rather than the lift. Spend time gardening, rather than watching TV. Go for a swim at the local pool. Combine this outlook with a workout program you devise from this book for a healthier lifestyle.

Your workout program should include cardio, strength and resistance training, as well as routines designed to increase balance and flexibility. The program should be performed for at least 30 minutes a day, three times a week. As you feel more comfortable, or need more of a challenge, increase the workout time to up to an hour. You can also increase the

number of days you do the workout. If you start training frequently, listen to your body – if you need a day off, take it to give your body time to recover.

Recommendation

It is highly recommended that you see your doctor prior to commencing an exercise program to ensure that it is safe for you to do so. If you have any pre-existing injuries, current injuries or a medical condition, it is not recommended that you start an exercise program unless you have a doctor's certificate (if you are going to be doing it in an exercise facility) or doctor's approval (if you are going to be doing it at home). If any exercises in this book cause you discomfort or pain it is recommended that you stop the exercise immediately and consult your doctor or a physiotherapist.

How to Use This Book

This book provides you with multiple exercises and stretches, and detailed instructions on how to perform each one correctly. It also gives you an idea of the benefits you will gain from doing an exercise or stretch, and outlines some tips on ways to get the most out of each one.

You will notice that each exercise has been given a level rating: beginner, intermediate or advanced. This indicates its level of difficulty. You should start at the beginner level and, as you improve your strength, core stability, range of movement and become increasingly confident in your ability, slowly progress to intermediate and finally to advanced. Once your program becomes routine, you will find that you are able to do a range of beginner, intermediate and advanced exercises. Just remember: the more regularly you exercise, the easier it will become.

This book also offers a range of different programs designed for varying fitness levels and goals. Firstly, you will need to choose your level and set some achievable goals for yourself. The programs are located at the back of the book, and contain several exercises, along with pictures, and the number of repetitions you should perform. They also have page numbers below the photographs so if you forget how to do a particular exercise you can flick back in the book.

The Different Components of Exercise

There are four major components of exercise: strength training, aerobic training, flexibility and balance. With each component there are many health benefits, but to feel the full benefits of an exercise program, all components should be included in a program.

Strength Training

Strength training is recommended for building strength and increasing bone density. It is also great for weight loss and cross training. It can be done with weights or even by using your own body weight. Strength training is ideal for anyone at any fitness level. It is effectively used in the prevention and management of multiple health conditions, including arthritis, osteoporosis, back pain, diabetes, obesity, high blood pressure and many others.

In the past, weight training tended to be only done by males, but now it is widely undertaken by both males and females of all ages and fitness levels. There is a misconception that women who lift weights will build too much muscle, making them look like body builders, or too manly. This is untrue. Females don't have the same muscle-building hormones as males, nor the body structure to support the muscles. Think about it: body builders lift really heavy weights at least five days a week, and eat huge amounts of food. They do both of these things for many years to get the muscles they have. If it's that hard for them to build even five kilograms of muscle, how could you build that much by having a balanced strength training program and eating a normal healthy diet? It simply cannot happen.

Remember too that muscles weigh more than fat, so by gaining 1 kilogram of muscle, and losing that in fat, you will look slimmer and shapelier. So in saying that, and understanding all the health benefits of strength training, there are only positives to strength training. Therefore you should get started as soon as you can.

Cardio Training or Aerobic Fitness

This form of training is normally described as involving exercise that increases your heart rate, and includes walking, running, bike riding, rowing and even circuit training. It is great for increasing fitness, lung capacity and endurance. Cardio training improves our lifestyles and makes daily tasks more enjoyable, such as walking to the letterbox to collect our mail or shopping for extended periods of time. Ultimately, cardio training will improve our quality of life.

Flexibility

Flexibility is the range of motion or movement through which our joints can move. When we move out of our range of movement, we are more inclined to injure or damage joints, muscles or tendons. As we age we lose flexibility. This is due to a process called 'fibrosis' whereby fibrous connective tissue takes the place of muscle fibres. Through exercise we can increase our flexibility and range of movement, and increase our blood flow, which reduces our chance of muscle injury. To maintain or improve our range of movement we need to reach our full range of movement at least once a day.

Motivation and Goal Setting

Motivation isn't something we're born with; it's something we develop and have to keep working on. Once an exercise program becomes routine, it's much easier to stay motivated. It takes at least four weeks of training before a program becomes routine. The first four weeks are very important and will normally determine whether you will continue training or lose your motivation. So to establish and help maintain good motivation levels, be as consistent as possible for six weeks. By then you should start seeing results and this, in turn, will help you stay motivated. Working out at the same time of the day, or the same days of the week, helps in this process. Make exercise an appointment that you can't miss. On a personal note, I write my workouts on my calendar with an allocated time. That way I know I have the time to do it, and can keep up my regular exercise regime.

Goal setting is an important component of motivation. When you reach your goals you will feel a sense of achievement and this will give you confidence in your ability to continue. When you start, don't be too ambitious. For example, if your goal is to lose 10 kilograms, break it up into smaller goals, for example: I am going to lose 3 kilograms in a month. When you achieve this, you will feel good, and motivated to continue. Then you can set yourself another goal to lose another amount of weight.

Ensure your goals are measurable as well as achievable. Having a goal such as, 'I want to increase my fitness' isn't measurable. However, having a goal of walking or jogging 2 kilometres is measurable. Putting measurable goals in place will ensure you stick with your exercise program and you'll be on your way to success.

Finally, rewarding yourself when you achieve a goal will also assist in maintaining your motivation. For example, tell yourself you will buy a new item of clothing when you achieve a 3- kilogram weight loss. You'll be surprised how much this contributes to you achieving the goals you set.

Getting Started

You have already taken the first step to fitness by reading this book and making the decision to start exercising. Now you just need to choose a time to exercise, find a place where you feel comfortable working out and decide whether you will exercise alone, or with a friend. Start off slowly. If you start out too hard too early you will tire and be less likely to continue exercising in the long term. In this book there are a range of program suggestions. Don't be afraid to change your program regularly. This will help you to feel challenged, maintain interest and keep motivated. Also ensure that you warm up sufficiently to avoid injury, and always stretch at the end of your workout – the stretches you do should correspond with the muscles you have worked.

Stretching for Flexibility

Before starting stretching, always warm up for at least 10 minutes. The muscles need to be warm to fully benefit from stretching, and it also reduces your risk of injury. Your body has a defence mechanism for preventing over-stretching: when your muscle reaches its range of movement the body sends a message to the muscle for it to contract very tightly, restricting the movement. This is called a stretch reflex.

The problem with this is that it is hard to increase your flexibility while the stretch reflex is resisting. So we rely on the golgi tendon organs (GTO), also referred to as autogenic inhibition, to facilitate the stretch or to relax the muscles enough to increase our range of motion. To initiate our GTO we can repeat the stretch several times holding for 20 to 30 seconds. This doesn't always work, so the sure way to improve our flexibility is to use a method of Proprioceptive Neuromuscular Facilitation (PNF) stretching. PNF stretching is a combination of static and isometric stretching. In English, just stretch your muscles as you normally would, then after holding the stretch for 10 to 15 seconds contract your muscles, pushing against the stretch. Hold this for 10 to 15 seconds, then relax and stretch further.

For example, when doing a chest wall stretch, push against the wall and contract your chest muscles. Hold for 20 seconds, then release. Attend the same stretch again; this time you should be able to stretch a little further. This will initiate the GTO and increase flexibility faster than any other stretch.

Breathing

The way we breathe is a very important part of our training. Breathing correctly while training will make it much easier for you, and help to ensure your muscles get the most out of each exercise.

A common mistake people make while training is to hold their breath. This restricts oxygen delivery to the muscles, and causes them to tire more quickly. Taking deep breaths provides the muscles with the oxygen they require. Breathing correctly means exhaling during the hardest part of the movement: if you were doing a squat you would breathe out on the way up. Always take deep breaths, ensuring you use the most of your lung capacity, delivering oxygen to the bottom of your lungs.

Breathing correctly will also help your core stability because it contracts your surrounding abdominal muscles. To ensure this happens, contract your abdominals while exercising. It also helps if you slow down your breathing while stretching because this relaxes the muscles, allowing them to lengthen.

Planning a Personalised Workout

We have many programs in this book suited to all levels of fitness, but if you want to plan your own workout there are some important things to take into consideration. When planning your workout it is wise to work from agonist to antagonist, or from front to back.

So if you do a chest exercise, follow it up with a back exercise. This will ensure you don't over-strengthen certain muscles, while leaving others weak, causing bad posture or rotation of a joint. You should also work larger muscle groups before smaller muscle groups. Your larger muscles would be your chest, back and legs. The smaller muscles are your arms, shoulders, abdominals and lower back.

If you train hard and feel tired, remember to give your body a rest day or two before repeating the program.

The Main Muscles of the Body

It is important that you can identify the muscles you are working in each exercise or stretch. By knowing the muscle or muscles you are targeting and identifying their function you can better understand how and why the exercise is conducted. By understanding this, you can tune into the muscles that you should be contracting when exercising or stretching.

Often when people exercise they are unable to feel the exercise working

The Body's Muscles and Their Location

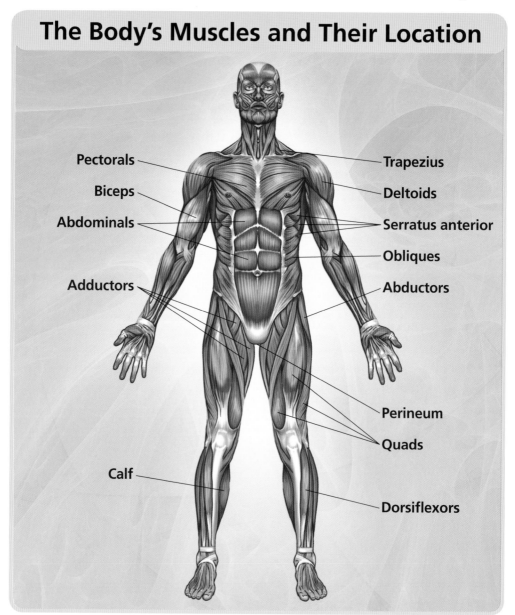

Pectorals

Biceps

Abdominals

Adductors

Calf

Trapezius

Deltoids

Serratus anterior

Obliques

Abductors

Perineum

Quads

Dorsiflexors

because they aren't concentrating on contracting the muscle properly. For example, when completing a bent row, the muscles contracting are the latissimus dorsi, rhomboids and lower trapezius. The action those muscles play together is drawing the shoulder blades together, so while pulling the dumbbells towards you, squeeze your shoulder blades together and contract the muscles in the back. Knowing the action and the muscle location will help you feel the exercise and receive its full benefits.

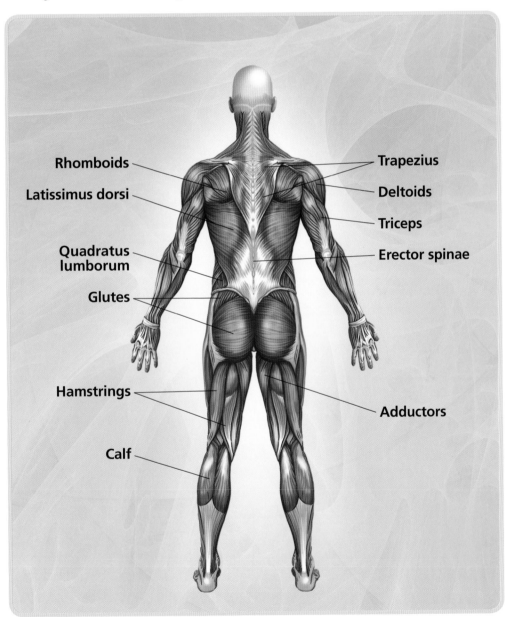

Rhomboids

Latissimus dorsi

Quadratus lumborum

Glutes

Hamstrings

Calf

Trapezius

Deltoids

Triceps

Erector spinae

Adductors

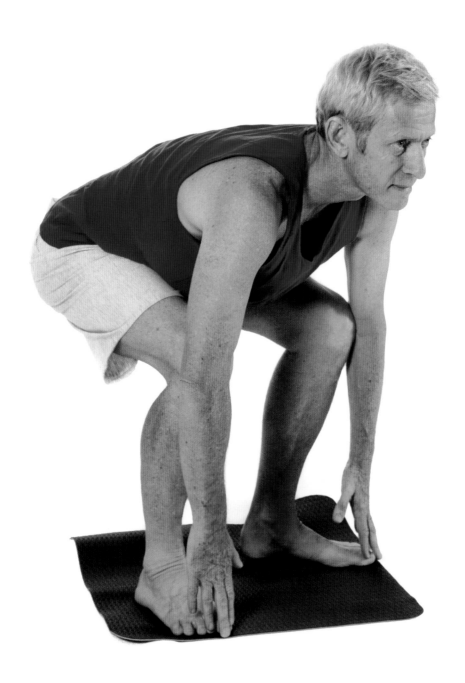

Chapter 2 Getting Warmed Up

Introduction

▸ Warming up is a very important part of any exercise program. It dramatically reduces the chance of injury during exercise and allows our bodies to slowly adjust in preparation for more intense exercise. The idea of warming up is to slowly increase body temperature and blood flow. It is a good idea to use your full range of movement in your warm-ups. This is achieved by rotating at the joints to their full range of motion. When warming up, it is suggested that you work from low to medium intensity – until there is a light sweat on your forehead. Do this for approximately 10 to 20 minutes. If it is a warm day you may only need 10 minutes of warm-up, while on a cooler day you may need longer. So, change your warm-up in accordance with the weather and how you are feeling.

Marching

Marching will help warm up your whole body and increase your heart rate. You can do it on the spot or while moving around. Marching is very similar to walking on the spot, only the movements are exaggerated. So swing your arms to shoulder height and lift your knees up so they are parallel with your hips.

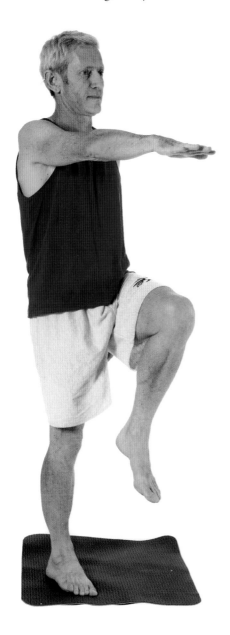
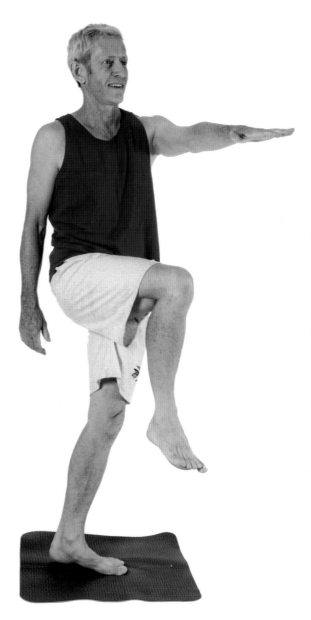

The Mexican Wave

Loosen up by bending down and touching your toes or knees then lifting your arms above your head in a wave motion. Repeat several times.

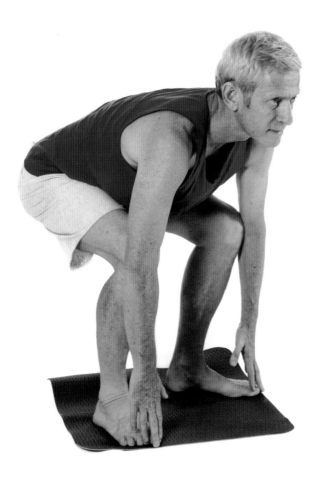

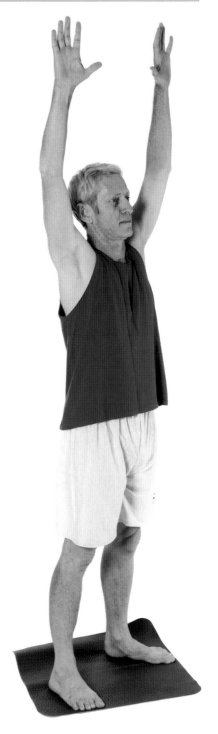

Side Stepping

Stand with your arms by your sides and your legs together. Then take a big step to the side with one foot. As you do this, bring your arms out straight in front of you at about shoulder height. Now bring your other foot to meet the one that you stepped to the side with; as you are doing this, bring your arms back down to by your sides. Then reverse the action by stepping to the opposite side, raising your arms out straight again, back to the position where you started. Repeat for 1 minute.

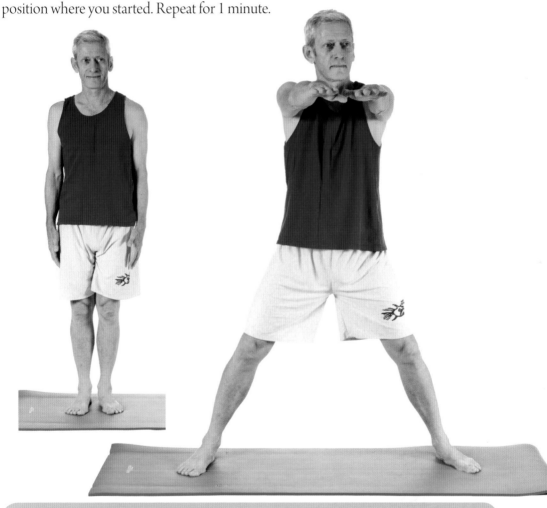

▶ Tip

To increase your heart rate, gradually increase the speed at which you are stepping side to side.

Ankles

Make circles with your ankles. Roll your foot around one way, then the other. Also move your foot up and down until it feels loose. Repeat on the other foot.

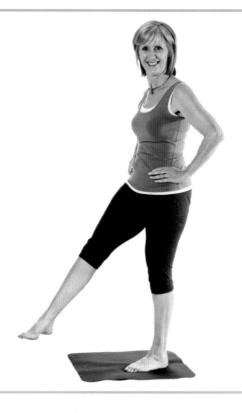

Joints

To increase the circulation to your muscles it is a good idea to rub your knees, elbows and any other joints that have poor circulation. This helps reduce joint discomfort during exercise. It is a good idea to repeat this several times a day.

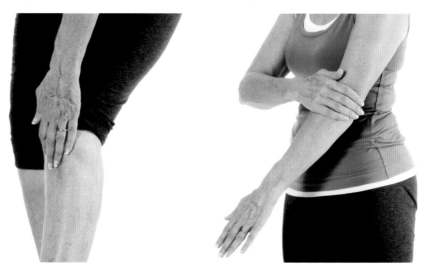

Arm Rotations

Stand upright with your arms out straight to your sides, like a clothesline. Turn your body from side to side, turning at your hips. Keep changing the direction of the circles as you go. Keep your feet stationary throughout the motions.

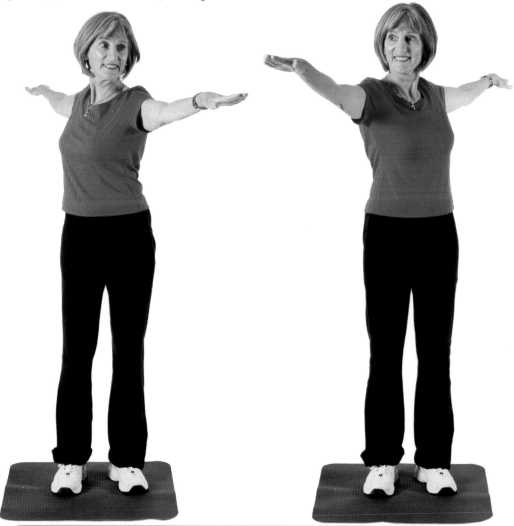

▶ **Variation**

Again put your arms out straight to your sides, then swing your arms across your chest and back to your sides again. Your arms should cross over in the middle.

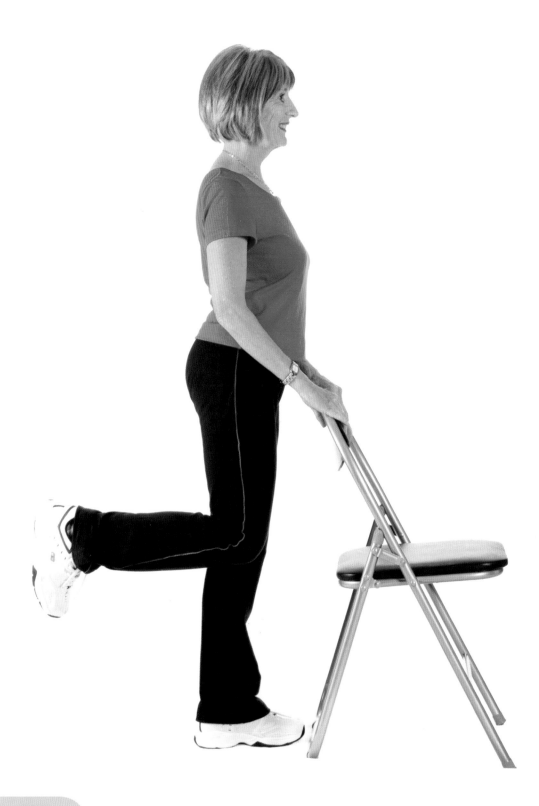

Chapter 3 Lower-Body Exercises

Introduction

▶ As we age, we tend to find it more difficult to sit, stand and bend and this is because we either have a decreased mobility in our joints, or a weakened or damaged muscle. Hence, it is very important to strengthen our legs in a functional way, to maintain independence, and lessen the need for assistance.

Another reason for working the lower body is that it increases circulation to our lower extremities, which aids with recovery and lessens the chance of injury and future medical problems.

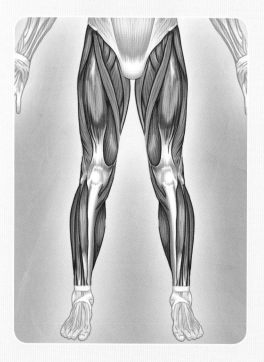
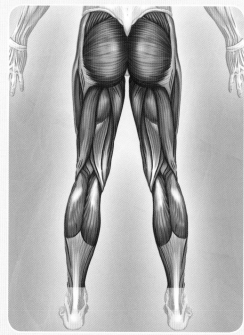

Squat

Level: Intermediate to Advanced

Benefits: Great for strengthening your legs and improving your balance.

Once you have warmed up, a squat is a terrific exercise to begin your lower-body workout. A squat is a great functional exercise, meaning it is a movement that we use in our day-to-day life. For example, every time you sit down, stand up or go to the toilet you are doing a squat.

Start with your feet shoulder-width apart and toes slightly pointing outwards. Cross your arms, placing your hands on your shoulders. Slowly bend your knees down to a 90-degree angle, ensuring your knees don't extend past your toes. Hold, and then slowly stand back up. Repeat 10 to 12 times.

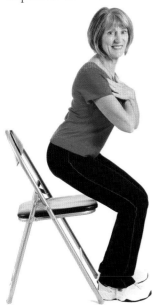

If struggling with technique, place a chair behind you and squat down as though you are about to sit – but stop just before your bottom touches the chair and then stand again.

Always remember that you should feel the pressure through your heels, not your toes. If you push through your toes, it could damage your knees over time.

▶ **Tip**

When performing a squat it is important to ensure you are always looking forward and holding your shoulders back.

Ball Squat

Level: Beginner

Benefits: This is a great exercise if you have back troubles. The ball supports your back as you squat. It is also good for improving your balance.

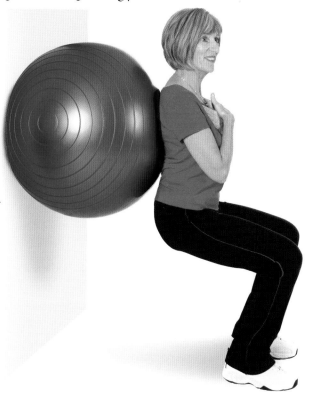

Place the ball against a wall at the lower curve of your back. Lean back onto the ball and allow it to support your weight. Place your feet shoulder-width apart and approximately half a metre out from the wall.

Inhale, then squat down until your pelvis and knees form a 90-degree angle. Hold for 5 seconds, and then slowly stand back up. Repeat this exercise 10 to 15 times.

▶ Tips

If you find you're pushing through your toes, or your knees are moving past your toes, lean further back on the ball and step away from the wall.

Ensure you don't lock your knees at the top of the movement.

▶ Variation

To further increase your strength, you can hold weights in both hands as you perform the exercise.

One-Leg Ball Squat

Level: Advanced

Benefits: This exercise is very good for balance and can improve your gluteal and quadricep strength.

Place the ball against a wall at the lower curve of your back. Lean back onto the ball and allow it to support your weight.

Lift one foot off the ground about 10 centimetres, and hold. Inhale as you ease down until your pelvis and knees form a 90-degree angle. (Ensure your knees don't go past your toes.) Then return to your standing position. This exercise can be repeated 6 to 10 times on each leg.

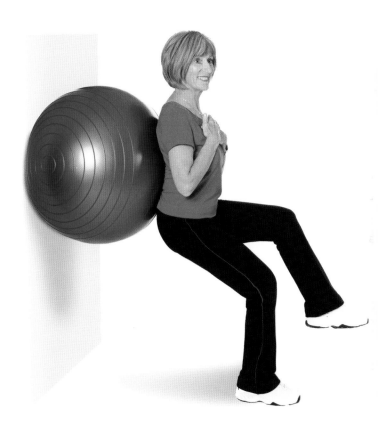

▶ **Tips**

Until you feel confident with the exercise, it is advised you use a chair to assist your balance.

Ensure your body stays upright – resist leaning to one side.

Standing Leg Curl

Level: Beginner to Intermediate

Benefits: The leg curl is a great strengthening exercise for your hamstrings, which are located at the back of your upper leg.

Stand behind a chair, using it for support. Exhale as you raise one leg off the ground behind you, ensuring you keep your knees together. Bend your knee up until it forms a 90-degree angle, hold for 2 seconds, then inhale as you release your leg back to its starting position. Repeat 10 to 20 times, and then change to the other leg.

▶ **Tip**

Contract your abdominal muscles in and up as you perform this exercise. This will help you maintain balance and provide support for your lower back.

Floor Leg Curl

Level: Beginner to Intermediate

Benefits: This exercise is easily performed. Being an isolated exercise, it targets your hamstring muscles.

Lie on the floor facing downwards, with your forehead on your hands, and thighs resting on a cushion or towel. Exhale as you bend your knee and draw your foot towards your buttock. Hold this pose for 2 seconds, then inhale as you slowly release your leg back to its starting position. Repeat 10 to 15 times, then change legs and repeat.

Leg Extension

Level: Beginner to Intermediate

Benefits: Strengthens your quadricep muscles and is an easy and safe exercise to do for all levels.

Sit on a chair. Exhale as you extend one leg out. Do not extend out until your knee locks. Draw your toes towards yourself. Hold for 2 seconds, then slowly release back to your starting position, ensuring your foot does not touch the ground. Repeat 10 to 15 times, then change legs and repeat.

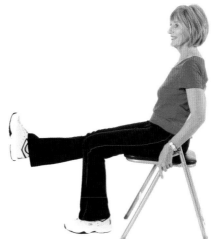

> ▶ Tip
>
> To make this exercise harder, add ankle weights.

Standing Leg Raise

Level: Beginner to Intermediate

Benefits: Strengthens the muscle on the outer side of your thigh.

Stand behind a chair using it for stability. Make sure you stand tall with good posture. Exhale as you raise your leg sideways as high as you can while maintaining an upright posture. Hold for 2 seconds, then inhale as you slowly lower your leg to its original position. Try not to let it rest on the floor as you lower it. Repeat this exercise 10 to 12 times on the same leg, then change legs and repeat.

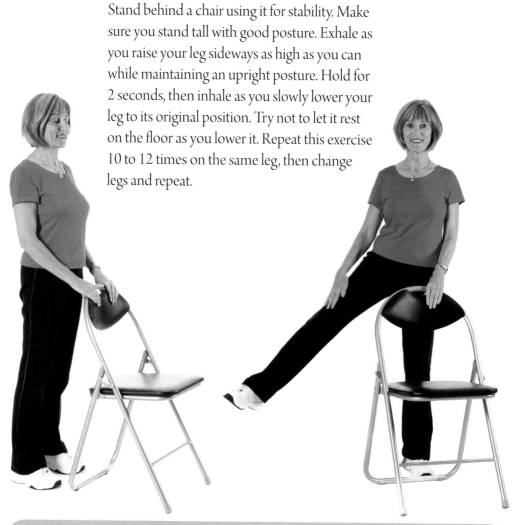

▶ Tip

Ensure you are standing upright through the entire movement. If you find your body tilting to one side, lower your leg.

Lying Leg Raise

Level: Beginner to Intermediate

Benefits: This is a safe exercise that isolates and targets your abductor and abdominal muscles.

Lie on your side with your elbow and forearm supporting your upper body and your other hand placed on the floor for additional support. Start with your feet and legs together , then exhale as you raise your leg to a comfortable but challenging height. Hold for 2 seconds, then inhale as you slowly return your leg to a few centimetres above your other leg. Repeat 10 to 15 times before changing to your other leg.

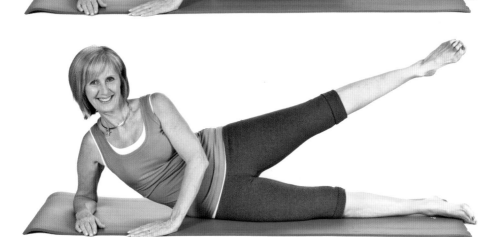

▶ Tips

Ensure your body doesn't roll backwards; support yourself with your hands on the floor.

Point your toes slightly downwards for greater muscle contraction.

Lunge

Level: Intermediate to Advanced

Benefits: Strengthens your hamstrings and your gluteal muscles. It can be a functional exercise, especially if you're a bowls player.

From a standing position, take a large step forward with one foot. Keeping a split stance, lift your chest up and keep your shoulders back. Squeeze your abdominal muscles. Now you're ready to start. While breathing in, bend your knees and lower your body weight down until your back knee is just off the ground or until you are comfortable. Hold for 2 seconds, and then exhale while lifting your body back to the starting position. Repeat 10 to 15 times and then change legs and repeat.

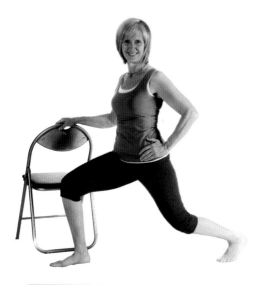

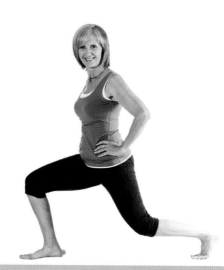

▶ **Tips**

Ensure your knee does not go past your toes on your front foot.

If needed, you can place your hand on a chair to provide extra support and balance.

▶ **Variation**

To increase intensity, you can hold a dumbbell in each hand. This will help improve your strength and balance.

Step-Up

Level: Beginner to Advanced

Benefits: Works your legs and increases your heart rate to help burn those kilojoules.

Stand in front of a step with your feet together. Lift your left foot up and place it on top of the step, then transfer your body weight onto your left foot. Now step up with your right foot. Both feet should now be next to each other on top of the step.

Now step back down off the step, left foot first. Transfer your body weight into your left leg, and then step your right leg back down to the floor. You should be back in your starting position. Repeat this exercise 10 to 15 times, then rest.

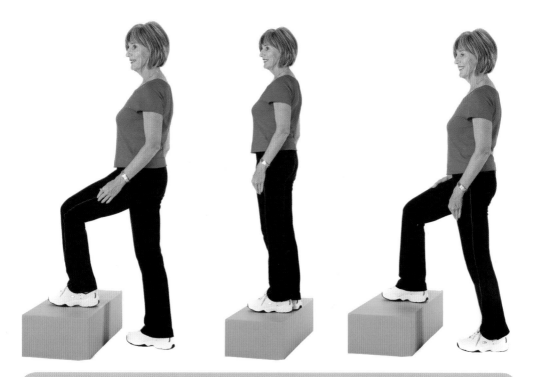

▶ **Tip**

Ensure you keep swapping the leading leg – if you step up 5 times with the left leg, then do the same amount on your right leg.

Knee Lift

Level: Intermediate to Advanced

Benefits: Can help to improve balance, knee-joint stability and strength in your legs.

Stand in front of a step with your right foot on the step and your left foot on the floor. Apply pressure through your left heel to push your leg up off the floor. Lift your left leg up, bending your knee and raising it until it reaches hip height. Hold this pose for 2 seconds, then bring your left leg back to its original starting position. Ensure the foot that is on the step stays there until all repetitions are completed. Complete 10 to 15 repetitions on each leg.

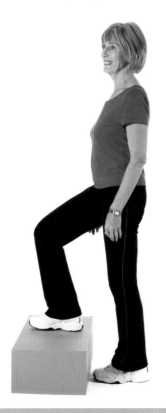 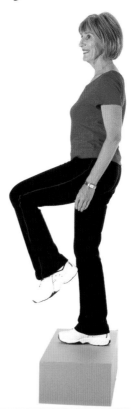

> ▶ **Tip**
>
> Ensure you step back off the step slowly so you don't over- or under-step and cause yourself an injury.

Sumo Squat

Level: Intermediate to Advanced

Benefits: Strengthens your inner thighs.

Place your feet about a metre apart – the wider your stance, the greater the muscle contraction. Look straight ahead, and have your shoulders back and down, and your chest up high.

Hold onto the end of one dumbbell with your two hands. Hold it between the middle of your legs. Inhale as you slowly bend your knees, lowering your body closer to the floor. Squat down until you feel the muscles in the inner sides of your legs contracting. Hold this pose for 2 seconds then exhale as you slowly raise your body back up to its original starting position. Repeat 10 to 15 times.

▶ Tips

Make sure you keep your back straight – looking straight ahead will help you achieve this.

Ensure that your knees don't extend past your toes when you are squatting – this will reduce the pressure through your knees.

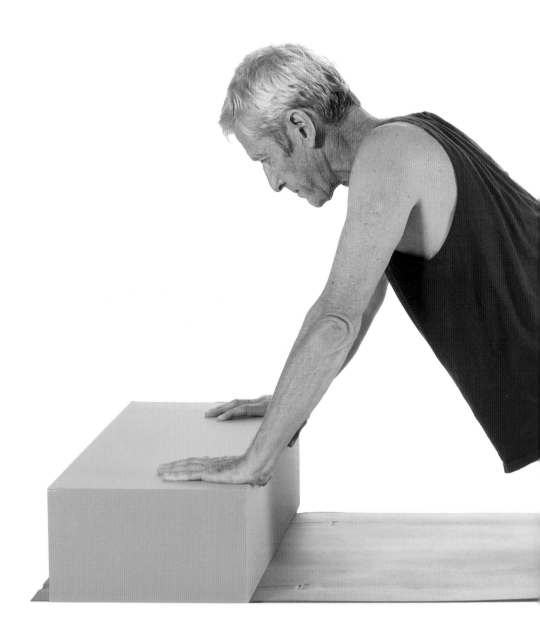

Chapter 4 About Chest Muscles and Training

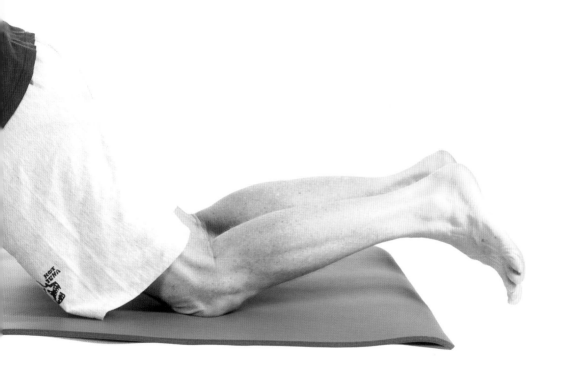

Introduction

▶ The chest is located at the front of the upper body, and
is considered one of the main muscle groups. It consists of
the upper pectoralis major and the lower pectoralis major.
Your chest is usually associated with the pushing movement.
Different exercises will work on different areas of the chest, so
it is important to perform a range of chest exercises to ensure
you work the upper, middle and lower aspects of your chest.

Working the chest muscles will help improve your upper-body
strength because the chest is a large muscle group. It will also
burn kilojoules as it works.

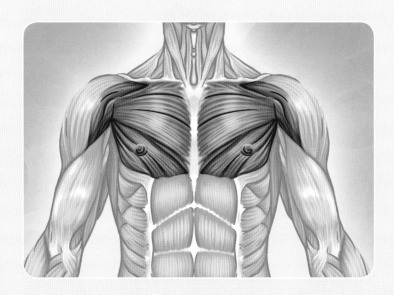

Wall Push-Up

Level: Beginner

Benefits: This is a good exercise to start building your chest, shoulders and arm strength. It's easy to do, you don't require any extra equipment, and you don't have to get down on the floor.

Stand in front of a wall so your fingertips are just a few centimetres away when both your arms are outstretched. Lean forward and let your palms touch the wall and take your weight, making sure your hands stay at shoulder height or lower. It doesn't matter if your heels lift off the floor when you're leaning forward.

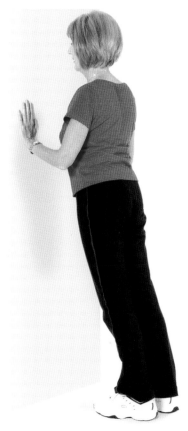

Inhale as you bend your elbows so that your upper body comes close to the wall, and your nose is nearly touching it. Exhale as you push yourself back until arms your are extended straight, then repeat 10 to 12 times.

> ▶ **Variation**
>
> To make the exercise a bit harder, and to work out your outer chest, you can place your hands further apart on the wall.
>
> When you have you hands closer together on the wall you are working your tricep muscles (back of upper arms) more. Variation will improve your strength and help you burn more kilojoules than if you were to continue doing the same exercise.

Push-Up on Toes

Level: Beginner to Advanced

Benefits: This exercise uses nearly all upper-body strength. If you have worked your way up to this exercise you will still find it a challenge, but not too uncomfortable. This exercise will build strength quickly.

Start from a kneeling position and lean forward so your hands touch the ground. Place them a little further than shoulder-width apart, in line with your chest. Now straighten your body so that it forms a straight line from head to toes. Your toes and hands should be the only thing in contact with the ground.

Contract your abdominal muscles, and inhale as you bend your elbows until your chest is a couple of centimetres above the floor. Then exhale as you push up, straightening your arms back to their starting position. Repeat 10 times.

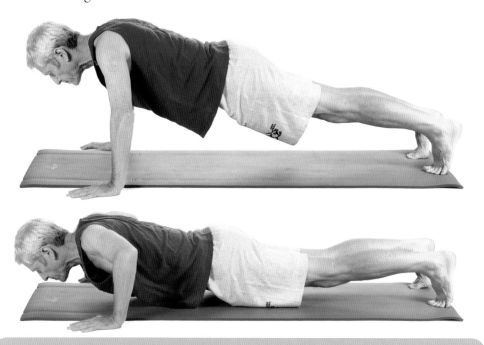

▶ Tip

To help avoid injury, try not to lock your elbows when you are performing a push-up.

Knee Push-Up

Level: Intermediate

Benefits: Increases strength, and works on your core strength and stability.

Kneel on all fours, keeping your knees together and hands shoulder-width apart. Keep your fingers pointing fairly forwards, and ensure you keep your body straight and your stomach tight. Bend your elbows and lower yourself down as far as comfortably possible, ensuring your elbows stay above your hands. Push back up while breathing out, then repeat 10 to 15 times.

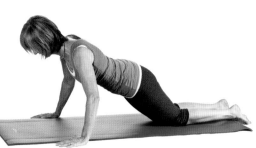

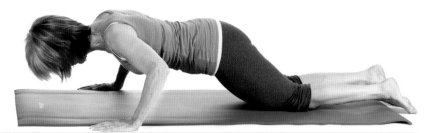

▶ Tips

If your knees are uncomfortable on the floor, you can place a folded towel or a small cushion under them.

Ensure you squeeze your shoulder blades together and draw them downwards – this will help maintain a good position for your upper back muscles. Contracting you abdominals will also improve your core strength.

Be sure to keep a line from your hands and chest. If there is an uncomfortable feeling in your shoulders, bring your hands slightly closer towards your knees.

You can start push-ups on a step and progress to the floor.

Knee push-ups can also be performed with your hands on a step or staircase. Doing this alleviates some of the pressure through the shoulders, and reduces the weight to be lifted during each push-up.

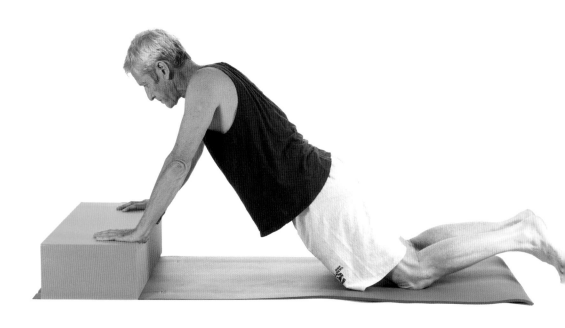

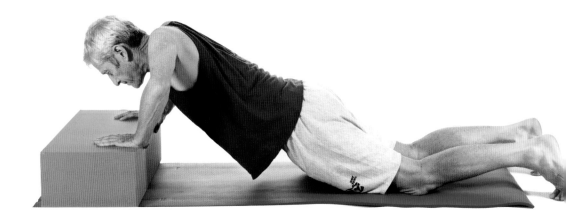

Chest Fly

Level: Beginner to Advanced

Benefits: This exercise strengthens your chest and the front of your shoulders.

Lie on your back with your knees bent and both feet flat on the floor. Hold a dumbbell in each hand. Exhale as you slowly draw the dumbbells together above your chest, with your palms facing each other. Draw your shoulder blades together and slightly bend your elbows.

Inhale, and then slowly lower your arms towards the floor, ensuring you keep the line of your chest and the same bend in your elbows. Lower to a few centimetres off the ground and stop. Slowly draw the dumbbells back together until they meet on top of your chest. Repeat 10 to 15 times.

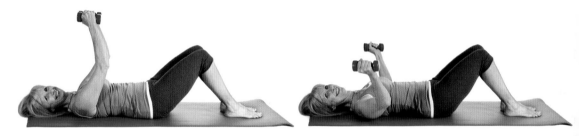

▶ **Tips**

Move slowly, as this reduces your risk of injury.

You should aim to complete each repetition over 6 seconds.

Try to squeeze the chest muscles together while working them, as this helps to achieve fuller muscle contraction through the exercise.

It is also beneficial to contract your abdominal muscles while performing this exercise because it helps improve core stability.

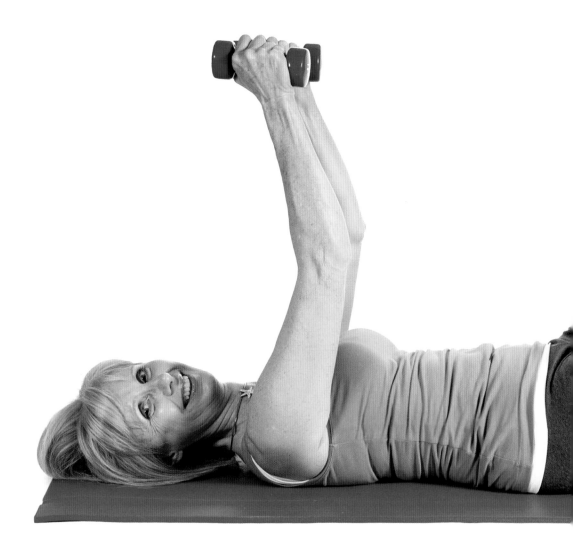

Chapter 5 About Back Muscles and Training

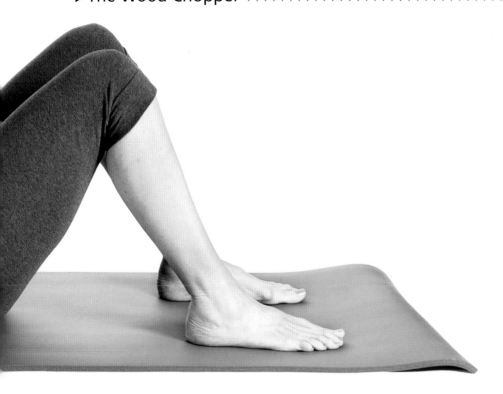

Introduction

▶ The back muscles can be categorised into five major parts: the erector spinae, latisimus dorsi, teres major, romboids and trapezius. These all have slightly different functions, but work together to enable the back to perform its job. The main movements of the back include the pulling movement, and drawing the shoulder blades together. So whenever you are pulling something up or pulling something down you will be utilising your back muscles. It is very important to strengthen the back, not just for strength, but to improve and maintain good posture.

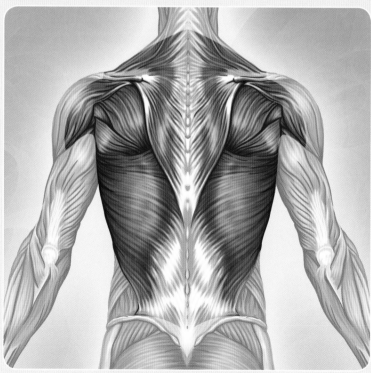

One-Arm Row

Level: Intermediate to Advanced

Benefits: This exercise will help to improve your mid-back, sides of the back and rear-shoulder strength.

Start with your right knee and hand on a step or stair, ensuring they are spread out wide. Now move your left leg out to your side for balance.

To start the exercise, hold a dumbbell in your left hand with your arm straight down. Look forward, and exhale as you draw the dumbbell up towards your hip bone, while squeezing your shoulder blades together and downwards. Your left elbow should be pointed up towards the ceiling. Hold for 2 to 3 seconds, and then inhale as you lower the dumbbell slowly. Repeat 10 to 15 times. When you have completed the desired amount of repetitions, change to the other arm.

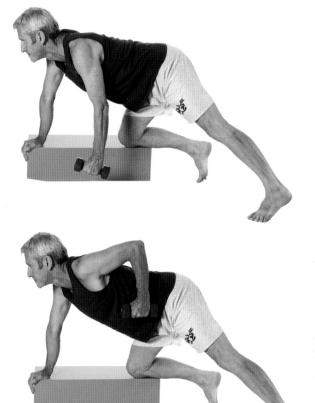

▶ Tips

Ensure your working arm remains close to your body as you lift and lower the weight. This will help work the targeted muscles.

Try to look forward while doing this exercise to assist you in maintaining good posture.

Squeeze your shoulder blades together to maximise the workload of the targeted muscles.

Bent Row

Level: Advanced

Benefits: This is a free-weight exercise that works on your abdominal muscles and core stability.

Start in a standing position with your feet shoulder-width apart, holding a dumbbell in each hand. Exhale and slowly squat down until the dumbbells reach your knees, then slightly straighten your legs keeping the dumbbells at knee height. Straighten your back and keep your chest up. Now pull dumbbells towards the middle of your abdomen and squeeze your shoulder blades together. Hold this stance for 2 seconds, then inhale as you slowly lower the dumbbells back to your knees and repeat.

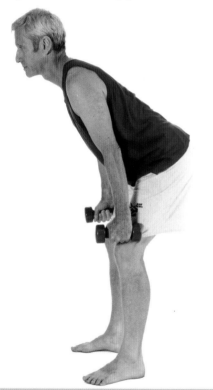 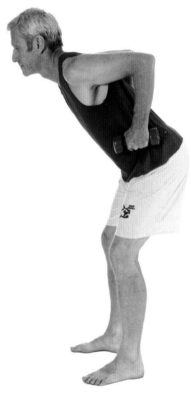

▶ **Tip**

Check your posture in a mirror to ensure your back is straight, not slouched!

Chair Row

Level: Beginner to Intermediate

Benefits: This exercise strengthens your back muscles safely and easily, because it is easier to keep a straight back while sitting.

Sit on a chair leaning forward, so your back is straight and your shoulders are back. Hold a dumbbell in each hand and lengthen your arms down straight by your sides. Exhale as you lift the dumbbells towards your abdomen and squeeze your shoulder blades together at the same time. Hold this pose for 2 seconds, inhale, then slowly lower the dumbbells down beside you to their starting position. Repeat 10 to 15 times.

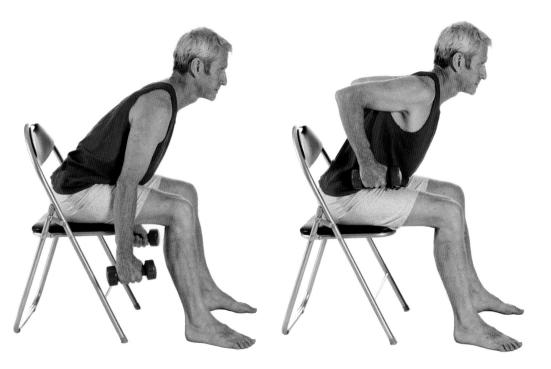

▶ Tip

Extend your chest forward as far as possible towards your knees while still keeping a straight back. This will maximise the use of your back muscles.

Reverse Fly

Level: Advanced

Benefits: This exercise strengthens the back of your shoulders, as well as your upper and mid-back.

Sit on a chair with your feet shoulder-width apart. Hold a dumbbell in each hand and lean forward in the chair. Maintain a straight back by pulling your shoulders back and looking at a spot on the floor about 1.5 metres in front of you. Keeping your body still, hold the dumbbells under your legs.

Exhale as you raise your arms out to your sides, keeping a slight bend in your elbows. Raise your arms to slightly lower than your shoulder height. Then inhale as you slowly lower the dumbbells back down to behind your legs. Repeat this exercise 10 to 12 times..

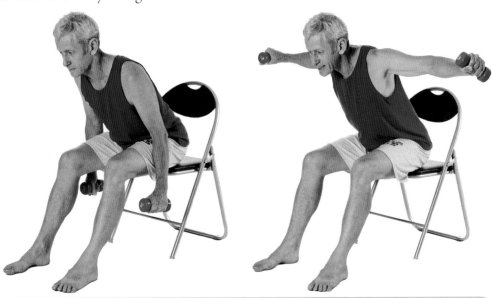

▶ **Tips**

Keep your arms in line with your shoulders during the entire movement and ensure your elbows are always positioned higher than you hands. Breathe out during the up phase.

If you find this exercise too difficult, gradually work your way up to performing it by practising one-arm rows.

The Wood Chopper

Level: Beginner to Advanced

Benefits: This exercise targets the side and mid-back muscles, and it also helps to strengthen and stabilise the muscles in the upper body which are involved in drawing your shoulder blades in together and down.

Lie on the floor with your knees bent and feet flat on the floor. Hold a dumbbell in each hand and bring up to above the centre of your chest. Draw your shoulders down and shoulder blades in together. Contract your abdominal muscles in and up and inhale.

Exhale as you slowly lower the dumbbells towards the floor from above your head – you will have to slightly bend your elbows as you do this. Stop just before the dumbbells reach the floor. Try to ensure you do not arch your back or slacken off on keeping your shoulders down when you do this.

Continue to exhale as you draw the dumbbells back to their starting position above your chest. Take a breath and repeat the exercise 10 to 15 times.

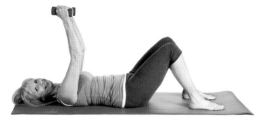 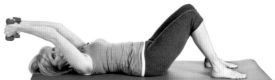

> **▶ Tips**
>
> This exercise feels really good if you've had a long day sitting at the computer with hunched shoulders, or your shoulders feel tense.
>
> Remember to draw your shoulders down to optimise the stretch and strengthen your back muscles.
>
> Try to avoid arching your back when you are lowering the dumbbells above your head.

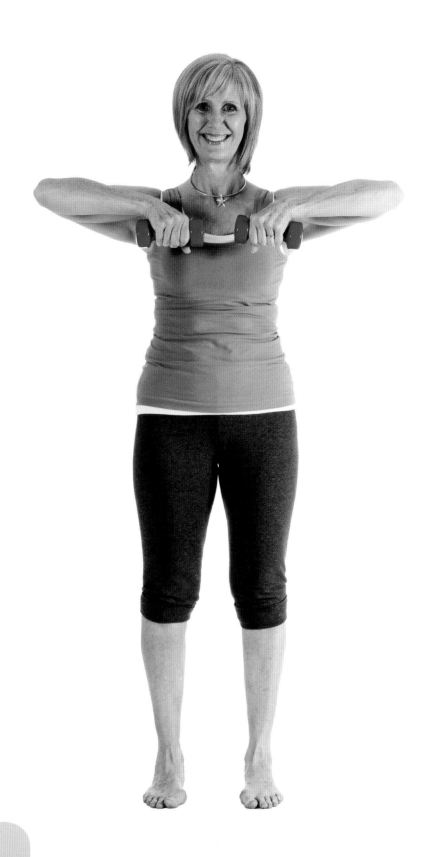

Chapter 6 About Shoulder Muscles and Training

Introduction

▶ Your shoulder muscles are also known as your deltoids. Their function is to mobilise and stabilise the shoulder joint, allowing you to rotate your arms within its range of movement. We also rely on the shoulder muscles to lift objects and reach up above our heads.

Whenever you do anything with your arms, it is working your shoulder muscles in some way. Therefore it is essential for us to train our shoulders to make day-to-day activities easier and less strenuous.

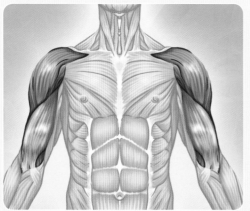 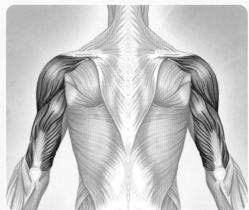

Shoulder Press

Level: Beginner to Intermediate

Benefits: Strengthens your shoulders while supporting your back.

Sit on a chair keeping your back straight, shoulders squared and chest high. Your feet should be placed flat on the floor at hip-width apart. Contract your abdominal muscles. Hold a dumbbell in each hand and raise them until they are in line with your ears. Exhale as you push the dumbbells above your head and touch them together directly above your head. Inhale as you slowly lower the dumbbells back to your ear-level. Repeat this exercise 10 to 12 times.

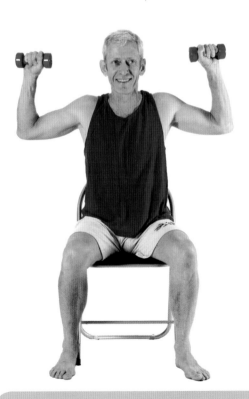
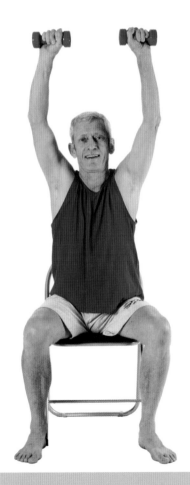

▶ **Tip**

Try to avoid arching your back, or pushing yourself back in the chair with your feet.

Muscle Press

Level: Intermediate to Advanced

Benefits: This exercise provides a full upper-body workout, and can assist in improving your co-ordination and upper-body strength. It is good if you have any shoulder problems because you don't have to rotate your shoulders.

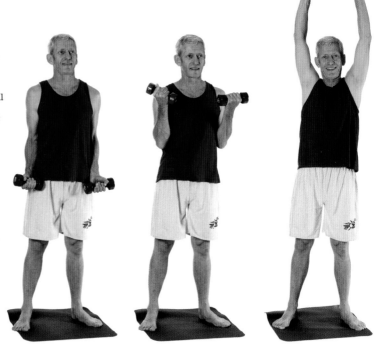

Stand tall with a dumbbell in each hand, and hands down by your sides. Exhale as you bend your elbows while lifting the dumbbells to your shoulders. Inhale, then exhale as you push the dumbbells up above your head, until your arms straighten out to an almost locked position. Then inhale as you slowly lower the dumbbells back down to your shoulders, and then back to your sides. Repeat this exercise 10 to 15 times.

▶ Tips

Try to keep your chest up and your body still as you perform the exercise.

Avoid a swinging motion with the dumbbells; instead try to do slow, steady movements.

Good concentration, posture and slow movements will optimise muscle contraction.

Upright Row

Level: Beginner

Benefits: Strengthens the backs of your shoulders, and is a safe and easy way to work your shoulders.

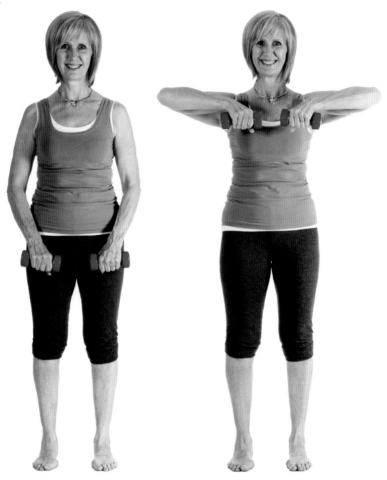

Stand upright with your chest high and shoulders drawn back. Hold a dumbbell in each hand, with the palms of your hands facing your thighs. Exhale as you lift the dumbbells up; ensure your elbows stay above your hands, and the dumbbells remain the same distance apart. Lift the dumbbells until your elbows reach shoulder height, remembering to keep your shoulders drawn downwards. Then inhale as you slowly bring the dumbbells back down to their starting position.

Repeat this exercise 10 to 12 times.

> ▶ **Tip**
>
> Keep the dumbbells lower than your elbows during the exercise. This will alleviate pressure from your shoulders, and ensure the target muscles are worked.

Single-Arm Lift

Level: Advanced

Benefits: This is a full-body exercise. It is also functional in that it mimics actions you do in your daily life. It increases your heart rate, and will burn kilojoules faster than many other exercises.

Stand with a dumbbell in one hand with a wide stance (further then hip-width apart), and place your other hand on your hip. Hold the dumbbell between your legs, then squat down keeping all the weight in your heels and maintaining a straight back.

Try to look at something high on the wall or on the ceiling. Once the dumbbell can touch the ground, exhale as you draw the dumbbell up with you and stand back upright.

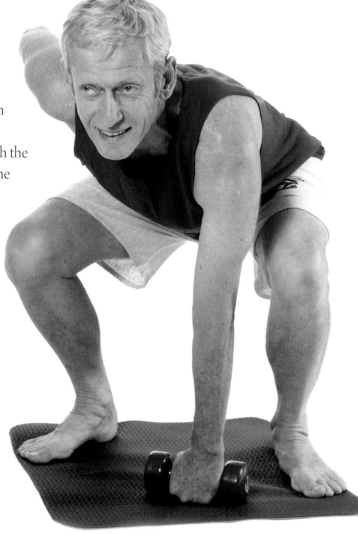

Inhale when the dumbbell reaches you shoulder, and exhale as you continue to push the dumbbell up above your head until your arm and knees are straight. Then inhale as you squat down again, bringing the dumbbell to the floor. Repeat this exercise 10 to 15 times.

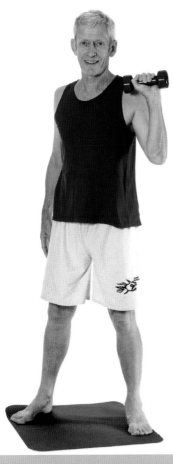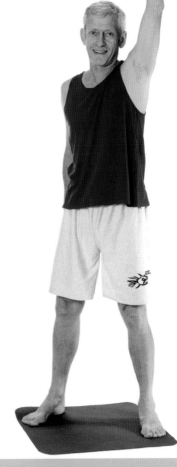

▶ **Tips**

Ensure you lift through your legs, without curving your back, so that you target the muscles that you are trying to work.

Try to look forward throughout the exercise. This will help you keep your back straight and assist in maintaining your balance.

At the top of the movement, try not to arch your back, because this will increase your risk of injury.

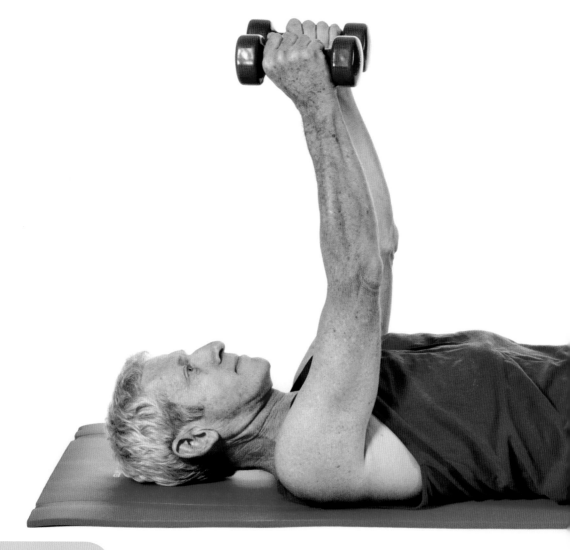

Chapter 7 About Arm Muscles and Training

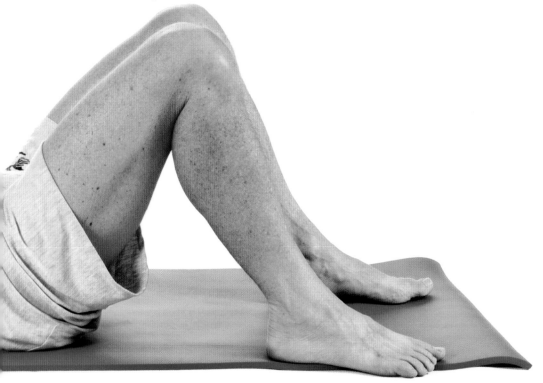

Introduction

▸ Your upper arm can be broken into two major components; the bicep, which is located in the front of the upper arm, and the tricep, which is located in the back of the upper arm. The function of these muscles is to flex and extend your arm. These muscles are used regularly on a day-to-day basis with all movements involving your arms.

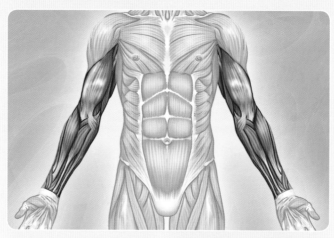

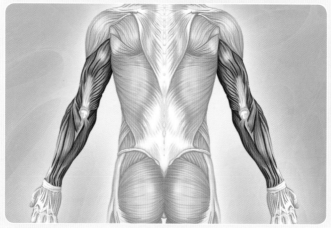

Bicep Curl

Level: Beginner to Advanced

Benefits: Strengthens your biceps, which are the muscles located at the front of your upper arms.

Stand in an upright position with your chest high and shoulders back. Place your feet hip-width apart, with your knees bent slightly. Hold a dumbbell in each hand, with the palms of your hands facing forward. Contract your abdominal muscles and draw your shoulders back and down.

Exhale and slowly lift the dumbbells toward your shoulders while keeping your elbows in the same position. Hold the dumbbells at the top of the movement for 2 seconds, then inhale as you slowly release them back down to their starting point. Repeat this exercise 10 to 15 times.

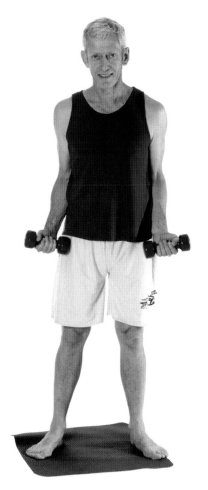
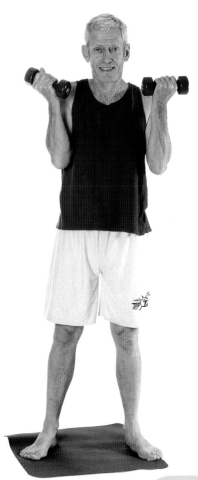

Hammer Curl

Level: Beginner to Advanced

Benefits: Strengthens the muscles of the sides of your upper arms, and helps improve upper-arm width.

Stand upright with your chest high, shoulders back and feet hip-width apart. Hold a dumbbell sideways in each hand, so that the insides of your hands are facing each other.

Exhale as you slowly bend your elbows, lifting the dumbbells towards your shoulders, while keeping your elbows still by your sides. Hold this pose for 2 seconds, then inhale as you slowly extend your arms back to the starting position. Repeat this exercise 10 to 15 times.

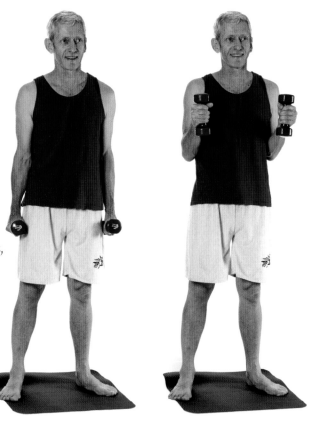

▶ **Tips**

Your palms should remain facing each other throughout the entire exercise.

Avoid any swinging motion; instead, slowly contract your muscles to gain the full benefit.

To break up the exercise routine, you can rotate between bicep curls and hammer curls.

Kickback

Level: Beginner to Advanced

Benefits: This exercise increases your muscle strength at the back of your upper-arms and your upper- and mid-back muscles.

Kneel on all fours. Line one elbow up directly under your shoulder, and have the other tight against your side. Ensure your back is straight, and draw your shoulder blades together.

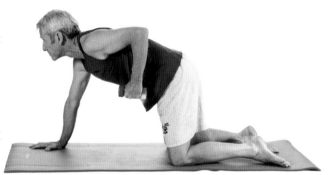

Hold a dumbbell in the hand that has the elbow tight up against the body. Exhale as you slowly extend that arm backward until it is completely extended.

Ensure you keep your elbow in line with your body, and then inhale as you slowly lower your arm back to its original position. Repeat 10 to 12 times.

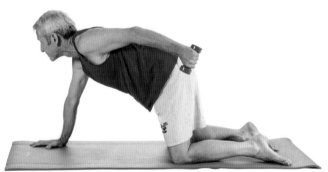

▶ **Tips**

Keep your working-arm elbow tight against your body to engage the correct muscles.

Concentrate on keeping your body square. If you start to swing, you may need to decrease the weight of the dumbbell you are lifting.

Tricep Extension

Level: Beginner to Advanced

Benefits: A great way to strengthen your tricep muscles.

Lie on your back with your knees bent and feet flat on the floor. Hold a dumbbell in each hand. Lift the dumbbells up until your arms are straight, directly above your shoulders. Pull your shoulders downwards, towards the floor. The palms of your hands should be facing each other.

Exhale as your slowly lower the dumbbells to beside your head. Rest and inhale, then exhale as you slowly lift the dumbbells back up until your arms are straight again. Repeat this exercise 10 to 12 times.

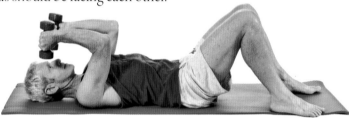

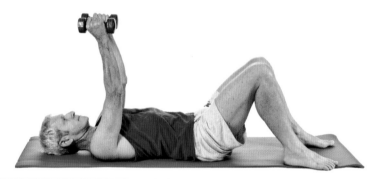

▶ Tip

Try to keep your elbows still and ensure you bring the dumbbells down slowly and in a controlled way to avoid hitting your head.

▶ Variation

You can also perform this exercise one arm at a time if you find using both arms too challenging.

Chair Dip

Level: Beginner to Advanced

Benefits: Strengthens the backs of your upper arms. It is a good functional exercise, because this action is performed several times throughout the day when getting up from your chair.

Sit on a chair with your hands placed on each of the chair's arms. Keep your chest up and shoulders down. Exhale as you lift your bodyweight off the chair using your arms; lift yourself up until your arms are nearly fully extended. Ensure your elbows stay behind your body and don't bend out to the sides.

Pause at the top of the exercise, and then inhale as you slowly lower yourself down until you are just a few centimetres from a seated position. Repeat this exercise 10 to 12 times.

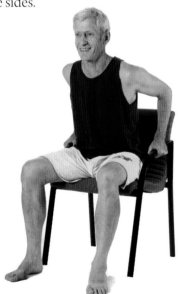

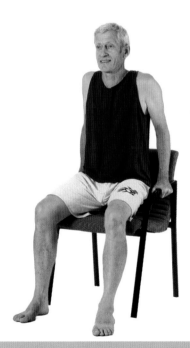

▶ **Tips**

Look forward throughout the exercise, and keep your chest up and shoulders back.

Really concentrate on keeping your elbows behind you, as this alleviates pressure on your shoulders.

Bench Dip

Level: Intermediate to Advanced

Benefits: Helps tone up and strengthen the backs of your upper arms, especially that area at the back of your arm where you are more inclined to hold body fat.

Start by sitting on a bench or step, with your feet straight out in front of you. Then place your hands by your sides, palms on the step, knuckles facing forward. Exhale as you lift your body weight up with your arms.

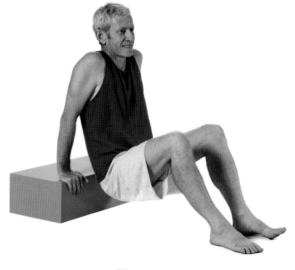

Slowly bend your arms, keeping your elbows still, and lower your torso towards the ground. Keep your body as close to the bench or step as you can, and inhale as you lower yourself down as far as comfortably possible.

Ensure your shoulders don't go lower than your elbows. Exhale as you lift yourself back up. Repeat 10 to 15 times.

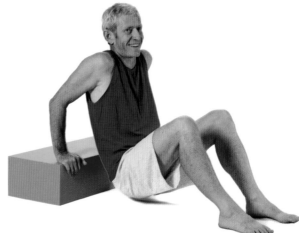

► Tip

To increase or decrease intensity, place your feet further or closer in front of you. (Further for increased intensity and closer for decreased intensity.)

Chapter 8 About Abdominal and Lower-Back Muscles and Training

Introduction

▶ The abdominals and the lower back breaks up into three major areas: your upper, lower and middle abdominals; your obliques; and your lower back. The main role of these muscles is to provide movement through your spine and torso, to lock the body into position and to correct posture. These muscles are designed to lock into an upright position when lifting heavy items and when walking.

If there is a weakness in any of these areas, it can cause back problems, pain or poor posture. That is why it is so important to strength train all muscle groups equally. If you do sit-ups for your abdominals and hovers for your lower back, this will provide equal strength training for the front and back of your body.

If one area is naturally stronger than another you will notice a change in posture. For example, if an individual has a really tight lower-back region, weak abdominals and forward hips, this can result in an arched lower back. This condition is referred to as lordosis, and is a spinal condition caused by tight muscles left for a prolonged period.

Chair Leg Lift

Level: Beginner

Benefits: An abdominal exercise that can benefit any level of fitness. It's easy to do, and can be done while sitting anywhere. Plus, you don't have to get down on the floor to do this.

Sit on a chair with your back straight and shoulders square. Place your feet together on the floor in front of you. Contract your abdominal muscles.

Exhale as you slowly lift both your legs off the ground. Hold them up for 5 to 10 seconds, remembering to breathe. Then relax, and place your feet back on the floor. Repeat this exercise 8 to 12 times.

▶ **Tip**

Concentrate on contracting your abdominal muscles, and not tipping forward in your chair. If necessary, you can hold onto the chair arms to assist you in maintaining balance.

Ball Crunch

Level: Intermediate to Advanced

Benefits: This exercise works more of your abdominal muscles than a traditional crunch. Using the stability ball will increase your balance, and provide your core muscles with more of a workout.

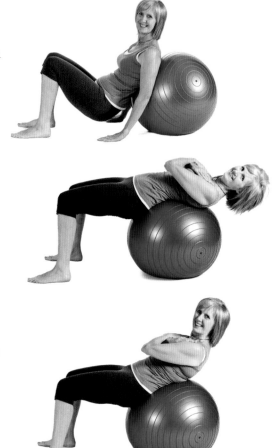

Sit on the floor with a stability ball up against your back, holding it behind you with your hands.

Slowly roll yourself back onto the ball, pushing yourself up onto it with your legs. The ball should sit under the arch of your back. Place your feet about hip-width apart and cross your arms on your chest. Ensure you feel safe and well-supported before you move onto the next component of the exercise.

Contract your abdominal muscles and exhale as you sit yourself up to about a 45-degree angle. Keep your shoulders squared while doing this. Then inhale as you slowly lower your back down onto the ball. Repeat this exercise 10 to 20 times.

▶ Tip

If you struggle with balance, you can place your feet up against the wall because this will help with stability. You can move your feet closer together for added difficulty or further apart for decreased difficulty.

Ball Twist

Level: Beginner to Intermediate

Benefits: This is a good exercise for your lower back and is good if you have lower-back problems because having your feet up on the ball alleviates pressure.

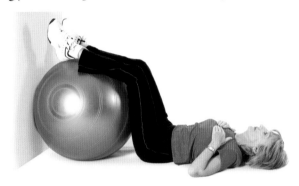

Place a stability ball up against a wall. Lie next to it on your back with your shoulders down. Engage your abdominal muscles as you bend your knees up and rest your lower legs on top of the ball. Exhale as you slowly lift your back up off the floor and extend you right hand out to touch the ball on the outer side of your left knee. Then inhale as you slowly lower yourself back down to the floor. Repeat using your opposite hand. Continue doing this for 10 to 20 repetitions.

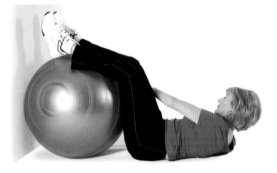

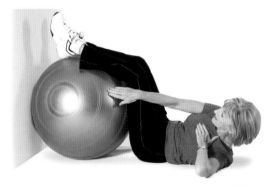

> ▶ **Tip**
>
> If you can't reach the ball with your hand just reach as far as comfortably possible – this is still beneficial.

Back Stabilising or Bird Dog

Level: Beginner

Benefits: Excellent for strengthening your lower-back muscles and for building your core stability.

Kneel on all fours, ensuring your back is straight, and looking towards the floor. Place your hands directly below your shoulders, with your hands facing forward. Make sure your knees are directly below your hips. Tighten your abdominal muscles and exhale as you slowly extend one leg until it reaches hip height, so that you form a straight line from head to toe. Hold this pose for 20 seconds; remember to breathe. Inhale as you slowly lower your leg back to its starting position. Repeat the exercise with your other leg. Remember to alternate sides. Repeat 6 to 8 times on each leg.

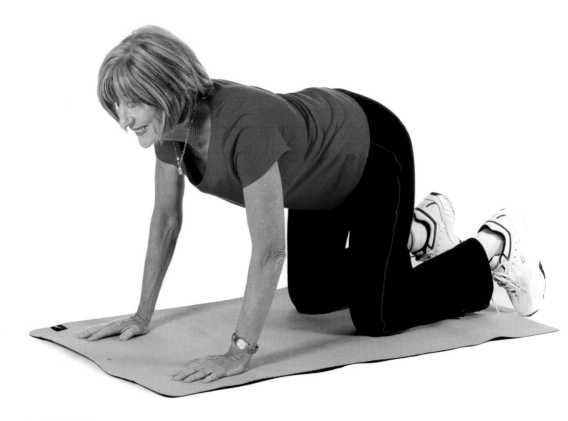

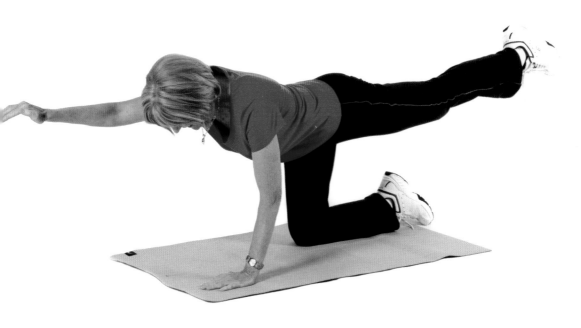

▶ Tips

Ensure slow movements and pause at the top of movements to ensure control and maximum muscle contraction.

Try to keep your shoulders and hips square. Your body will want to twist, but avoid it because it will stop the target muscles from working to their full potential.

▶ Variation

Kneel on all fours, ensuring your back is straight and abdominals are squeezed. Exhale as you extend one leg out, making the same straight line from your fingers to your toes. Then outstretch your opposite arm. Try to keep your shoulders down while doing this. Hold for 20 seconds, remembering to breathe, and then inhale as you slowly draw your outstretched arm and leg back in to their starting positions. Alternate from one side to the other, and repeat for 6 to 8 times.

The Plank

Level: Beginner to Advanced

Benefits: Provides a workout for your upper and lower core muscles, as well as the muscles in your chest, shoulders and arms.

Start by getting down on all fours. Place your hands together on the floor, with your fingers facing forward. Your elbows should line up underneath your shoulders. Draw your shoulders down and ensure your head is in line with your back. Extend your neck, but remain looking down at the floor below you.

Tightly squeeze your abdominal muscles and draw your pelvic-floor muscles up, which strengthens your lower core, and provides increased support. Slowly extend your right leg back, with your toes underneath your heels.

Slowly extend your left leg back in line with your right leg. Straighten your legs, including your knees. Hold this pose for approximately 3 breaths, concentrating on maintaining tight abdominal muscles – this will help keep your back straight, and prevent it from sagging.

To resume the starting position, slowly lower your knees to the floor one at a time. Have a rest, then repeat this exercise a further 3 times. When performing this exercise again, try to hold the pose for as long as comfortably possible.

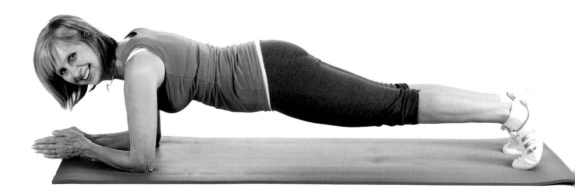

The Plank with Leg Raise

Level: Intermediate to Advanced

Benefits: This exercise will further strengthen your core muscles, as well as working your gluteals and hamstring muscles.

Get yourself into the plank pose. Again tighten your core muscles, and then exhale as you slowly raise your right leg about 30 to 50 centimetres off the floor. Hold this pose for a few breaths, then inhale as you slowly lower your leg to its original starting position. Then change legs. Repeat this exercise 4 times, changing legs on each occasion.

To resume the starting position, slowly lower your knees to the floor one at a time.

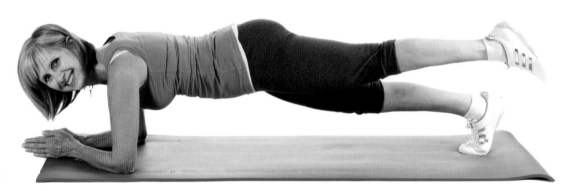

Sit-Up

Level: Beginner to Advanced

Benefits: Strengthens and firms your abdominal and core muscles.

Lie on your back with your knees bent upwards and the soles of your feet flat on the floor. Now place your hands on your thighs. Exhale as you use your abdominal muscles to lift your shoulders and upper back off the floor; lift up until your hands slide up to your knees. Then inhale as you slowly lower yourself back down to the floor, ensuring your shoulders don't rest on the floor. Repeat this exercise 10 to 20 times.

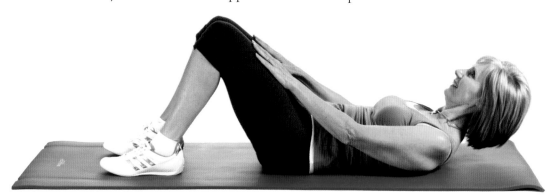

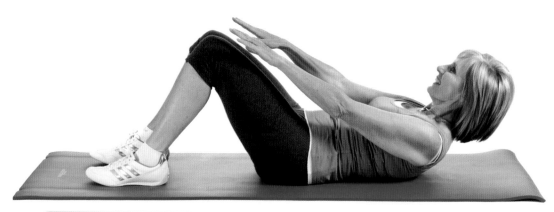

▶ **Tips**

To keep your neck from hurting, find a spot or mark high on the wall or on the ceiling to look at while completing the sit-ups. This will keep your head and neck still thoughout the movements.

Pelvic Thrust

Level: Beginner to Advanced

Benefits: This exercise can strengthen your abdominals, lower-back, hamstrings and gluteal muscles. It is also good for improving your pelvic-floor muscles.

Lie on your back with your knees bent and the soles of your feet flat on the floor. Both your feet and knees should be about hip-width apart. Place the palms of your hands flat on the floor beside you.

Exhale as you push firmly down through your hands, arms, shoulders and especially your feet, to raise your hips off the floor as high as possible. Hold the pose at the top for 2 seconds, then inhale as you bring your body back down to the floor. Repeat this exercise 10 to 12 times.

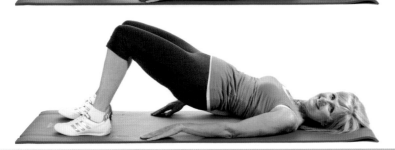

▶ **Tips**

You can perform this exercise as part of your warm-up because it incorporates most of the large muscle groups.

To work the gluteal muscles more, you can lift your toes off the ground, and push through your heels.

Looking in a mirror can also help to ensure good form.

Be careful not to push pressure through your neck or head – keep the pressure going through your arms and shoulders.

Knee to Elbows

Level: Intermediate to Advanced

Benefits: This exercise works your abdominals, as well as increasing your core stability and upper-body strength.

Start on all fours, ensuring your hands are directly under your shoulders. Lift your body off the floor – the only thing making contact with the floor is your toes and the palms of your hands. Exhale as you bend one knee up past your chest and try to reach the same-side elbow with your knee. Maintain a straight back and keep your hips square. Once you have either touched your elbow with your knee or reached as close as you can, inhale as you place your foot back to its starting position. Repeat this exercise 10 to 20 times, alternating legs.

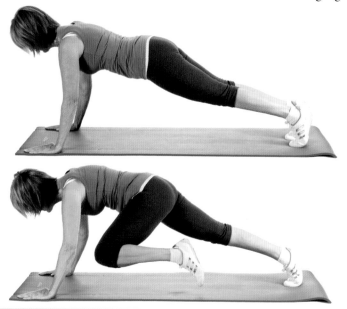

> ▶ **Tips**
>
> Try to keep your back as straight as possible. You may not reach all the way to your elbow, but go as far as comfortably possible.
>
> If needed, you can place your hands up on a step; this will help alleviate some of the pressure through your shoulders.

Side Hover

Level: Intermediate to Advanced

Benefits: Helps strengthen and stabilise your core muscles.

Lying on your side, place your forearm and elbow underneath your shoulder. While keeping your feet together, lift your body up so that just your feet and your forearms are touching the ground. Ensure you keep a straight line from your toes to your head. Now, with your other arm, point to the ceiling directly above your shoulders. This will keep your torso square. Hold for as long as possible, then release and change sides and repeat.

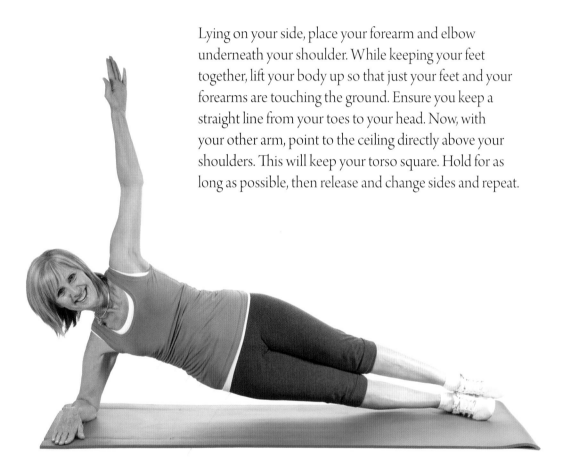

▶ **Tips**

Ensure you keep your arm pointing to the ceiling because this will help you to keep your body square.

Really squeeze the muscles located at the sides of your hips, because this is where you are most likely to lose form when doing the exercise.

Bicycle Crunch

Level: Intermediate to Advanced

Benefits: According to research this exercise is far more effective than a regular abdominal crunch. It targets both your rectus abdominis muscles and your external oblique muscles. These are the muscles that are most involved in toning your abdominals and trimming down your waistline.

Lie on your back with your hands by your ears and your knees bent up to your chest. Squeeze your abdominal muscles, and draw up the floor of your pelvis. This will help engage your lower core muscles. Draw your shoulders down towards the floor and inhale.

Exhale as you lift your shoulders off the floor, while curving your upper spine.

Start to twist your upper body, bringing your right elbow towards your left knee while extending the right leg. Hold this pose for 1 to 2 seconds, remembering to keep your shoulders off the floor.

Then twist your upper body the other way, making your left elbow twist towards your right knee and extending your left leg. Repeat 10 to 15 times each side.

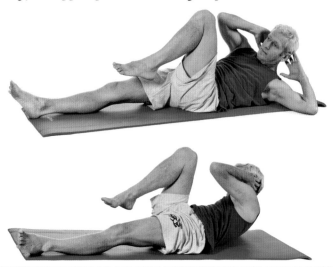

> ▶ **Tip**
>
> Keep your upper spine curved and shoulders off the floor throughout the entire exercise. This will optimise contraction of your abdominal muscles.

Jack Knife

Level: Advanced

Benefits: A great way to work your abdominal muscles while also increasing your heart rate, so great for burning off those kilojoules.

Lie on your back with your legs and arms extended straight out. Contract your abdominal muscles and exhale as you bring your upper body and knees up so they meet in the middle. Ensure your shoulders are up and off the floor when your knees meet your chest, and make sure you contact the palms of your hands with the floor. Slowly relax, then extend your arms and legs back out to their starting position. Repeat 10 to 12 times.

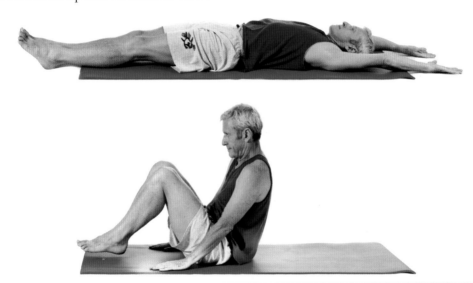

▶ **Tips**

The harder you hit the floor with your hands, the greater the abdominal muscle contraction, and the more intense the exercise will be.

Avoid bringing your knees in too quickly because this will make it much harder for you to lift your shoulders off the floor.

By sitting up slightly before bringing in your legs, you will find the exercise much easier.

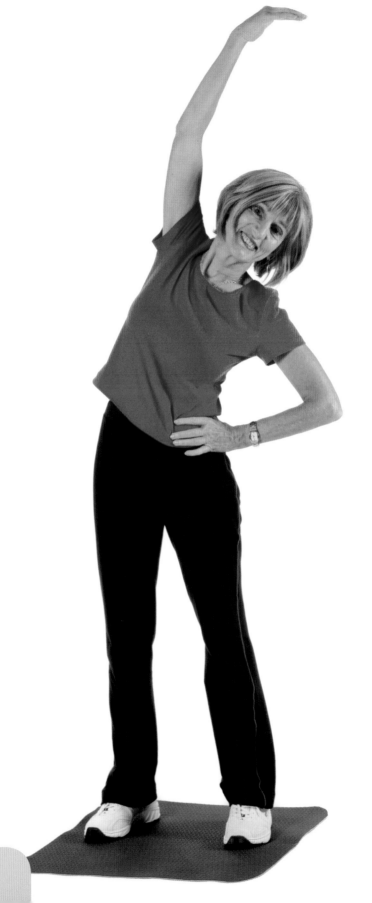

Chapter 9 Upper-Body Stretches

Introduction

▶ Stretching is a very important aspect of strength training. As you train, your muscles may tighten up, reducing your range of movement. After training, stretching helps your body to recover and reduces your risk of sustaining an injury. Stretching will also help maintain and potentially improve your flexibility and mobility. Furthermore, stretching your upper-body muscles correctly will help facilitate good posture and minimise curved shoulders and a hunched back.

Pull-Across Shoulder Stretch

Benefits: Stretches your mid- and upper-back muscles, and the back of your shoulders. This exercise can also be done in the seated position.

Standing tall, bring one arm across your chest, and place the hand of your other arm on the elbow. Draw the elbow towards your body, ensuring the arm across your body is straight. You should feel this stretch though the shoulder. Hold for 20 to 30 seconds, then release and change arms.

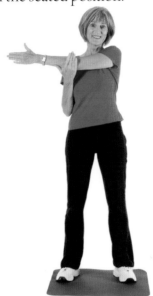

Shoulder Two-Handed Stretch

Benefits: This exercise can be done at any time throughout your workout if you need a break. It also stretches the top of your shoulders and chest.

Stand tall, keep your chest up and shoulders square. Draw your shoulders down and squeeze your shoulder blades together. Join your hands together behind your back making a fist; this will lock your shoulders into position. Hold the stretch for 20 to 30 seconds, then release.

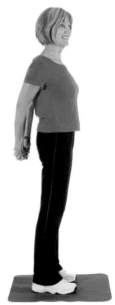

Back Stretch

Benefits: Stretches your upper back and shoulders.

Stand approximately half a metre away from a wall and face towards it. Place both your hands as high as possible on the wall, keeping your half-metre distance. Now apply pressure through your hands onto the wall and push your chest downwards. You should feel the stretch through your sides and under your arms. Hold this stretch for 20 to 30 seconds, then release.

Chest Wall Stretch

Stand on a slight angle with a split stance (one leg forward and one leg back), next to a wall. Place one of your elbows and forearms against the wall, and the palm of your hand on the wall. Ensure you form a straight line from your shoulder to the elbow that is up against the wall. You can place your other hand on your hip. While keeping your elbow still, rotate your body away from the wall until you feel your chest stretch. When you have reached the desired stretch, hold for 20 to 30 seconds, then release and change arms.

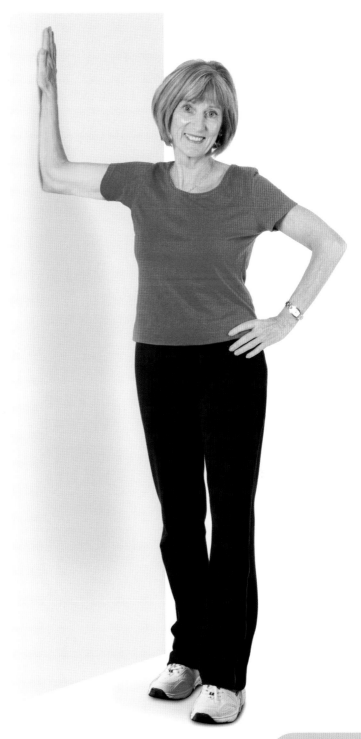

Child's Pose

Kneel on the floor with your knees hip-width apart. Lean forward, so your nose is nearly touching the ground. Rest your arms by your sides with the palms of your hands facing the ceiling. Relax through the body and exhale. You can slowly take 5 to 6 deep breaths throughout the stretch to help you feel relaxed.

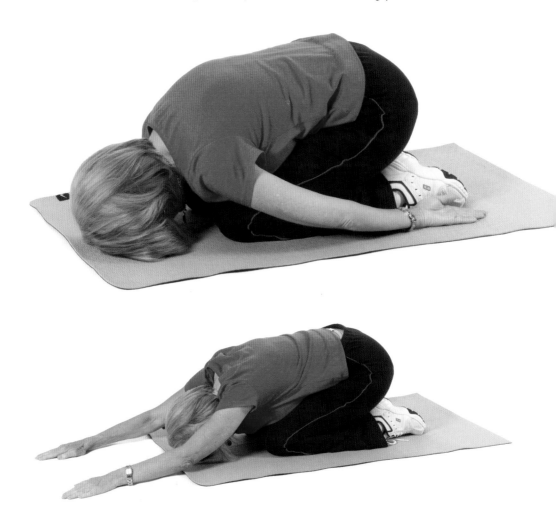

▶ **Variation**

Place your arms out in front of you with your palms facing down. Keep relaxed through the stretch and breathe slowly.

Foetal Roll

Start by sitting on the ground. Bring your knees up to your chest and hug your legs. Ensuring you relax your back and shoulders, roll backwards from your buttocks onto your back. Then roll forward again to resume the sitting position. Repeat this stretch 8 to 12 times.

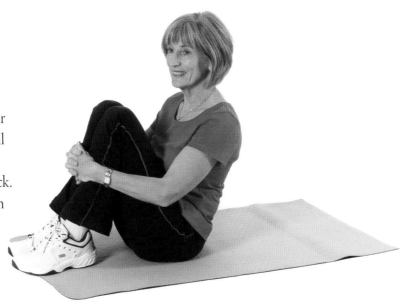

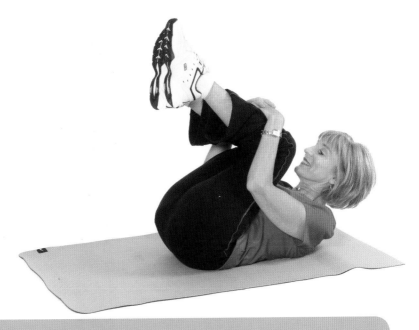

> ▶ **Tip**
>
> Ensure you don't roll back too far – if your neck touches the ground when rolling, you are rolling too far back.

Leaning Stretch

Stand tall with your feet about hip-width apart. Place one hand on your hip and the other hand up above your head. Now reach with the hand that is above your head towards the opposite side of your body. Lean across until you can feel the stretch through your side. Ensure you keep your body square and chest up. Hold the stretch for 20 to 30 seconds, then release and repeat with your other side.

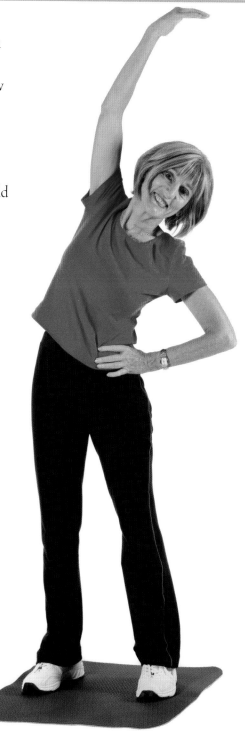

Morning Stretch

Kneel on all fours. Arch your back downwards towards the floor, keeping your shoulders square, and drawing your shoulder blades together.

Look up at the ceiling as you exhale and drop your thighs towards the floor. You should feel the pressure release from your back, and the stretch through your abdominal muscles. Hold this pose for 10 to 20 seconds, and then slowly release yourself back to the starting position. This stretch can be repeated several times.

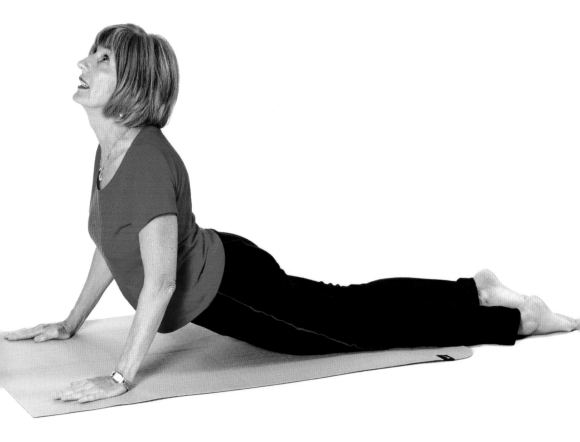

▶ Tip

Do this stretch very slowly, and relax through the stretch to feel its full benefit.

Trunk Rotation

Sit on a chair with your feet flat on the floor about hip-width apart. Keep your chest high and shoulders back and down. Twist your upper body towards the left, bringing your right hand across the front of your body and placing the palm of your right hand on the outer side of your left knee. Then use your right arm to further twist your body to your left – this will assist in stretching your lower-back muscles. Hold this pose for 20 to 30 seconds, then release and twist to your opposite side.

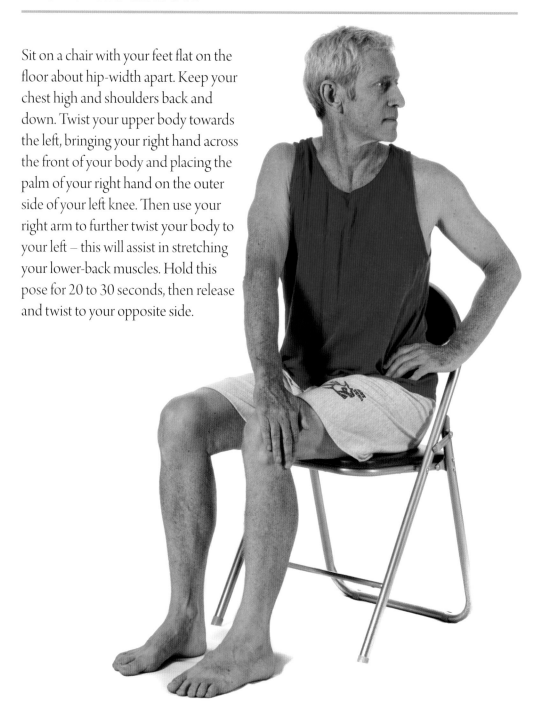

Bicep Stretch

Stand tall with your shoulders square. Hold one arm out straight in front. Bring your other hand across so the palms of your hands meet together. Keep the arm that is facing upwards straight, and push your fingers down towards the floor with your other hand. You should feel the stretch through your forearm and bicep. When you feel the stretch, hold for 20 to 30 seconds. Then change to repeat on your other arm.

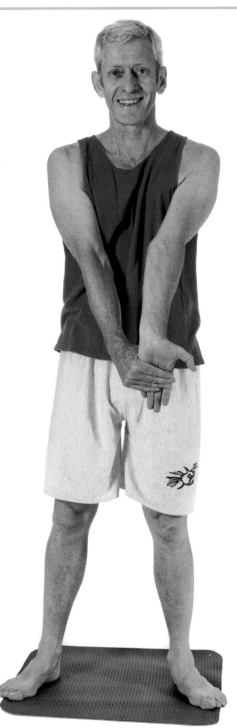

Lying Twist

Lie flat on your back with your arms spread out to your sides. Bend both your knees up and raise your feet off the floor so that your knees are directly above your hips.

Exhale as you slowly twist your lower body to one side, aiming for your legs to touch the floor beside you. Don't worry if you can't reach, just stretch to your ability. Once you have achieved this, slowly bring your legs back so your knees are again directly above your hips. Proceed to then stretch your other side.

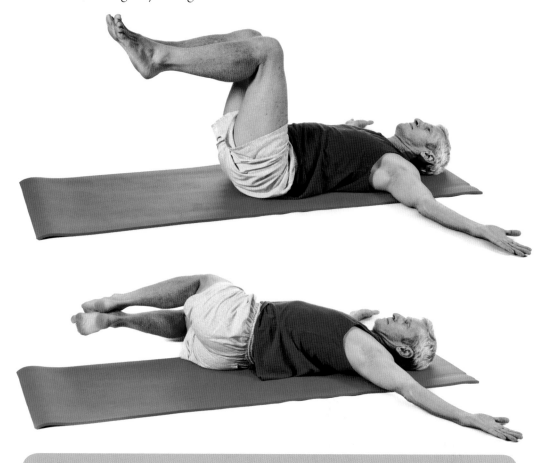

▶ **Tip**

Avoid lifting your shoulders off the floor as much as possible. Looking in the opposite direction to the way your legs are rotating may also help you keep your shoulders on the floor.

Double Bicep Stretch

Standing tall, start with your arms by your side. Draw your hands out behind you and then twist your hands, rotating your thumbs inwards and away from you, until they will go no further. When this is achieved, hold for 20 to 30 seconds, and release.

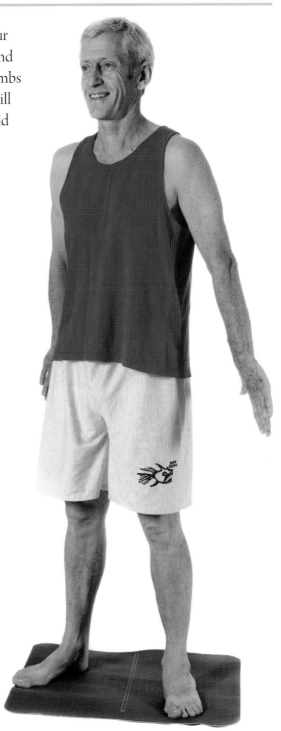

Tricep Stretch

Benefits: Provides a good stretch to your tricep muscles and also increases your shoulder mobility.

Place one hand over the top of your head, and touch your opposite shoulder. Your elbow should be pointing up towards the ceiling. Then place your other hand on your elbow and slowly pull your elbow closer towards your head, until you reach your stretching point. Try to keep your shoulders square, back straight and head facing forward. When you have held this stretch for 20 to 30, slowly release, change arms and repeat.

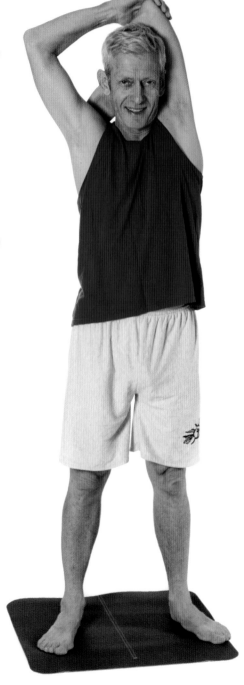

Chapter 10 Lower-Body Stretches

Introduction

▶ We use our lower body throughout most of the day, which can result in muscle tightness and fatigue. Continued use of your lower-body muscles increases your risk of muscular injuries, such as muscle tears and strains. Therefore, it is imperative to regularly stretch these muscles. Regular stretching will help you to recover, maintain flexibility and help you to continue undertaking your day-to-day activities with a reduced risk of injury and fatigue.

Gluteal Stretch

Benefits: This is a good stretch to loosen up your gluteal muscles. These are an often overlooked muscle group when stretching, but can get very tight.

Sit on the ground with one leg straight and the other bent and placed over your straight leg, so as to make a bridge. Then hug your bent leg and draw it to your chest until you can feel the stretch. Hold for 20 to 30 seconds, then change legs and repeat.

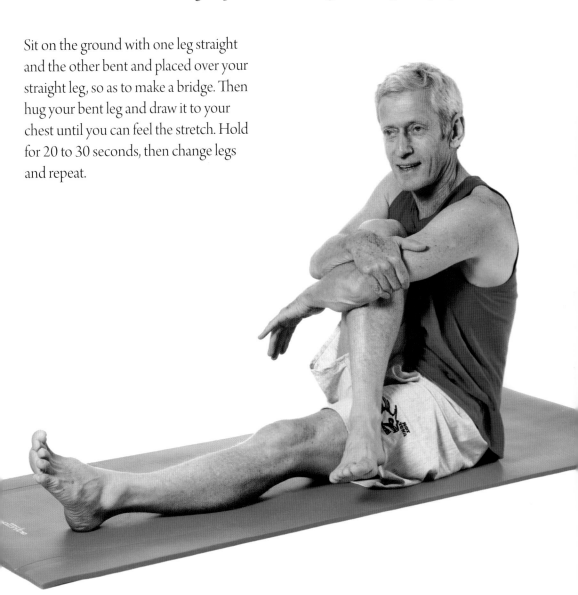

Downward Facing Dog

Start on all fours. Place you hands on the floor, further out than your shoulders. You feet should be about hip-width apart. Then straighten both your arms and legs. You buttock should be poking up in the air, and your body should form the shape of a pyramid. Now push pressure through your hands and through your heels. Hold this stretch for 20 to 30 seconds, then release.

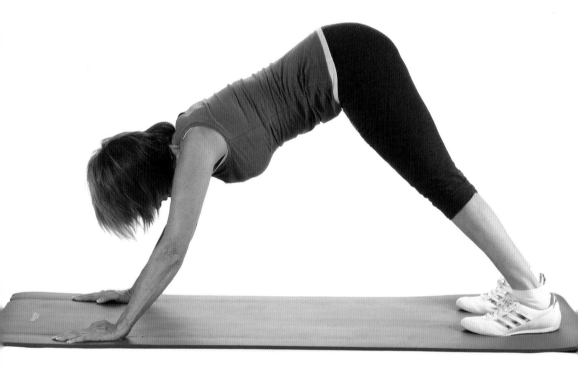

▶ Tips

Ensure you straighten the upper body because the lower-back region has a tendency to curve. To prevent this from happening push harder through your heels and engage your quadricep muscles.

Be careful to not put pressure through your shoulders. If you find this is occurring, tilt your head forward and look at your hands.

Standing Calf Stretch

Benefits: Helps lengthen your calf muscles and alleviate pressure from your Achilles tendons which are located at the backs of your heels.

Start in an upright position with a split stance – one leg forward, one leg back. The wider your stance, the greater the stretch. Ensure both your feet are facing forward. Slightly bend your front leg, but not past your toes. Push the weight through your back heel ensuring a constant pressure (no bouncing). Hold the stretch for about 20 seconds then swap legs.

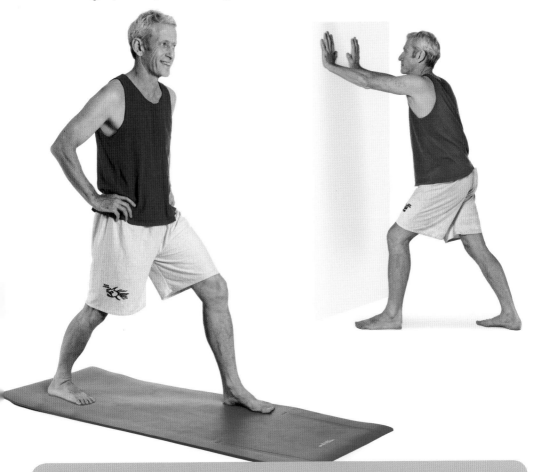

▶ **Variation**

You can place your hands on a wall for extra support and a greater stretch in your working calf.

Calf Wall Stretch

Benefits: Great for those who already have flexible calf muscles because this stretch is intense, stretching more of your calf muscles, and more deeply.

Stand in front of a wall in an upright position. Place the ball of your foot on the wall, about three-quarters of your shoe length high from the floor. While keeping your heel on the ground, bring your knee closer to the wall, pushing against it with the balls of your feet. Hold for 20 to 30 seconds, then release. Swap legs and repeat.

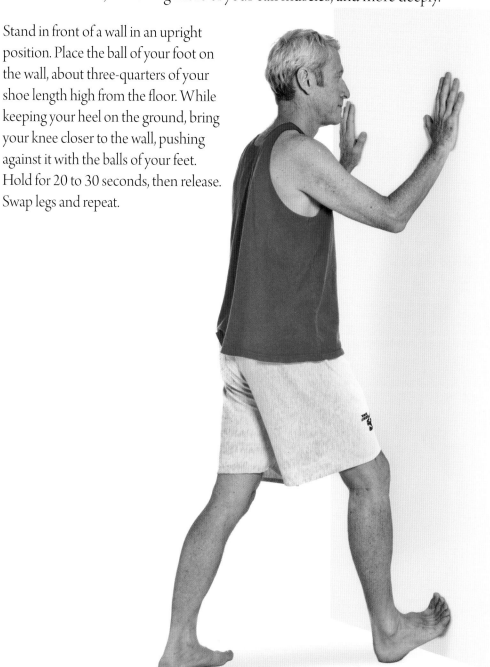

Standing Quadricep Stretch

Stand in an upright position looking forward. Place all your weight on your right foot, then bend your left knee up and draw your left foot back towards your buttock. Grab hold of your left foot with your left hand. Remember to keep your knees together. Bring your left foot closer towards your buttock until you can feel the stretch, then hold for 20 to 30 seconds. Repeat the stretch on your other leg.

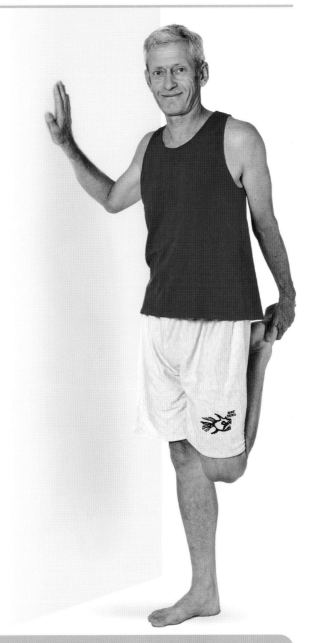

▶ **Tip**

You may need to place one hand on the head of a chair or on a wall to assist in stabilising yourself.

Assisted Quadricep Stretch

Stand in front of a chair. Place your left foot on the chair, with your right leg supporting your body weight. Now bend your support leg and bring the resting foot closer to your buttock. Keep lowering your body by bending your supporting leg until you get the desired stretch. Hold the stretch for 20 to 30 seconds. Repeat the stretch on your other leg.

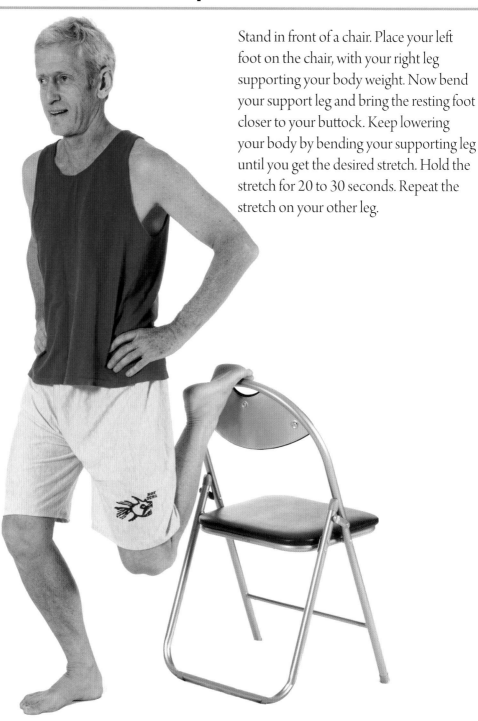

Lying Quadricep Stretch

Lie on your right side using your right arm to support your head. Bend your left leg up towards your buttock. With your left hand grab hold of your left foot if you can. While keeping your body in a straight line, pull your foot towards your buttock to increase the stretch. Ensure your knees stay together throughout the stretch. Hold for 20 to 30 seconds, then roll onto your other side and repeat on your opposite leg.

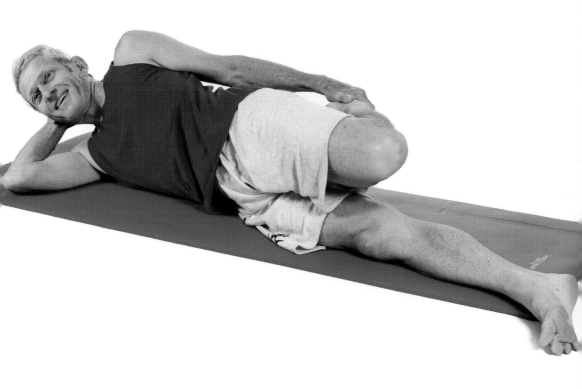

Seated Hamstring Stretch

Sit on the edge of a chair with both feet hip-width apart, and flat on the floor. Straighten out one leg in front of you. Now with your same-side hand, reach down towards your toes. If you can't reach your toes, that's fine – just reach out until you can feel the stretch in your hamstrings (behind your upper leg). Hold for 20 to 30 seconds, then release. Change sides and repeat.

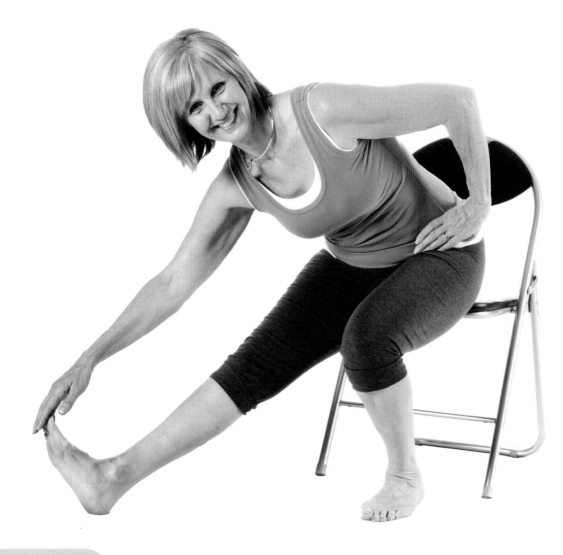

Standing Hamstring Stretch

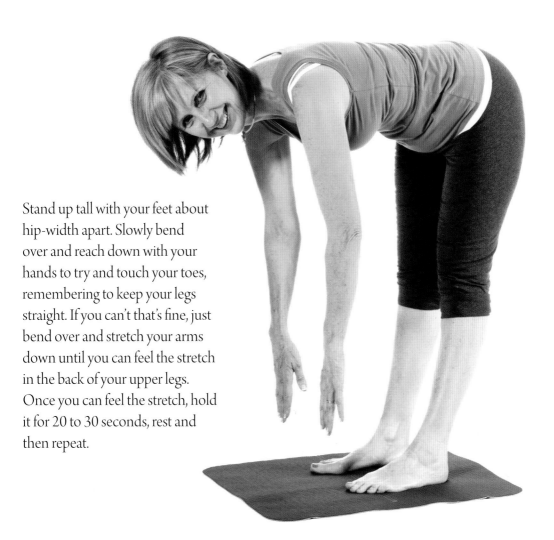

Stand up tall with your feet about hip-width apart. Slowly bend over and reach down with your hands to try and touch your toes, remembering to keep your legs straight. If you can't that's fine, just bend over and stretch your arms down until you can feel the stretch in the back of your upper legs. Once you can feel the stretch, hold it for 20 to 30 seconds, rest and then repeat.

▶ **Tip**

Ensure your movements are slow and controlled. Don't bounce to reach your feet as this may cause injury.

Floor Hamstring Stretch

Sit on the floor with both your legs straight out in front of you. Gently bend your left leg up and rest the sole of your foot on the inside of your right thigh, then relax your left leg down, so your leg is resting on the floor. Keeping your right leg out straight, lean forward and try to touch your toes. If you are unable to, just reach as far as comfortably possible. When you can feel the stretch, hold for 20 to 30 seconds, and then change legs.

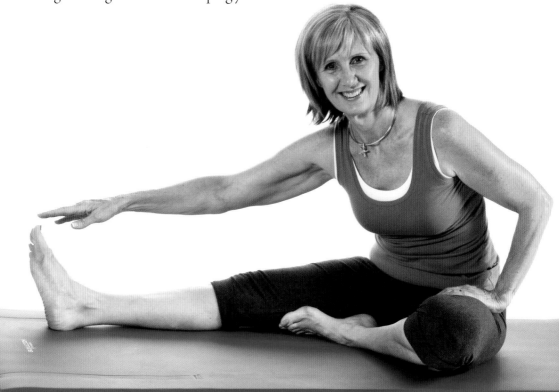

▶ **Tips**

Ensure you hold the stretch and don't bounce the stretch as this can cause injury.

Take your time – if it is causing you pain ease off a little, as you may be over-stretching.

Standing Groin Stretch

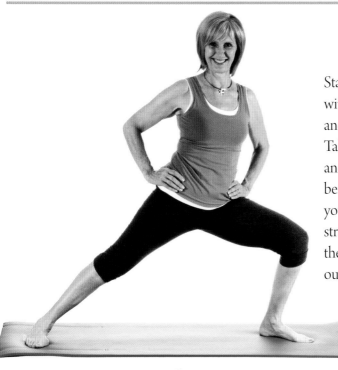

Stand in an upright position with your shoulders square, and your hands on your hips. Take one big step to the side, and straighten one leg, while bending your other leg. Ensure you keep your toes on your straight leg pointed forward and the toes on the bent leg turned outward 45 degrees.

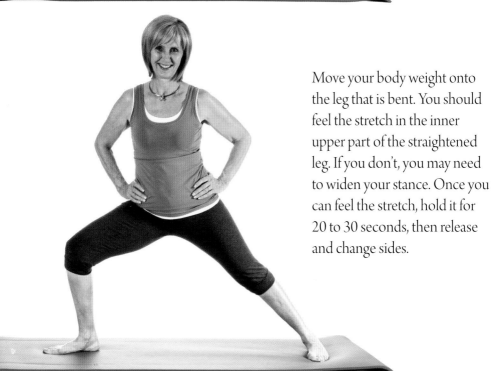

Move your body weight onto the leg that is bent. You should feel the stretch in the inner upper part of the straightened leg. If you don't, you may need to widen your stance. Once you can feel the stretch, hold it for 20 to 30 seconds, then release and change sides.

Floor Groin Stretch

Sit on the floor with a straight back and square shoulders. Bring the soles of your feet towards each other and draw them as close to yourself as possible. Secure the soles of your feet together by clasping your hands around them. While holding your feet, push your elbows down on your knees. This will intensify the stretch. Hold the stretch for 20 to 30 seconds, then rest.

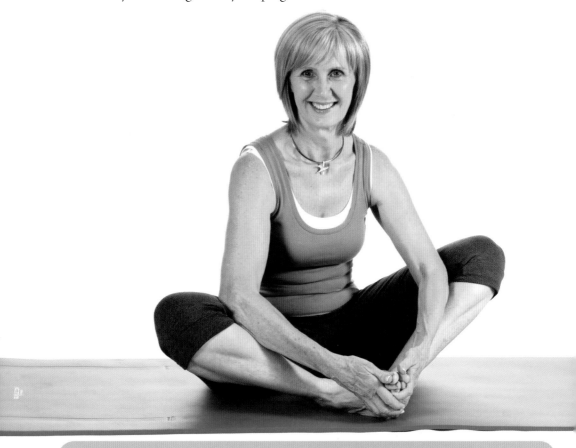

▶ **Variation**

Sit on the floor with your legs spread out to the sides as far as possible, while maintaining straight legs. Then lean your body forward and place your hands out on the floor in front of you. Hold this stretch for 20 to 30 seconds, then rest.

Chapter 11 Balance

Introduction

▶ Balance is one of those things most of us take for granted, and don't really think about. It is described as core stability, and involves remaining relatively still when your surroundings are unstable. While doing these exercises, deep muscles surrounding your joints and bodily structures tighten to support you. As they strengthen, your balance improves.

It is important to maintain and improve our balance no matter our age or our fitness level, as it can reduce the risk of, and even prevent, accidents and falls. As we age, balance becomes increasingly important due to the fact that we are more likely to sustain a serious injury when we fall. Furthermore, our recovery phase from injuries and falls can be prolonged, and affect our independence and mobility. Hence, it is crucial to incorporate balance into our exercise regime.

Balance exercises should be done as often as possible, every day if you can. You can achieve greater core stability and balance through stability-ball exercises, yoga, tai chi, Pilates, strength training and balance exercises.

Proprioceptive

It is a good idea to practise balancing with your eyes closed (proprioceptive balance) while holding onto something like a secure chair. This is much harder than balancing with your eyes open, and you should only attempt it when you are completely comfortable and feel safe. Always ensure that your hand is on a chair for that extra bit of security and support.

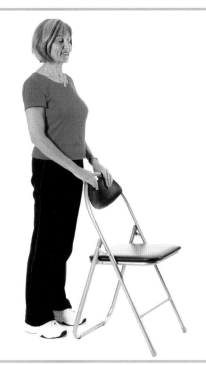

Chair Balance

Level: Beginner to Intermediate

Benefits: Increases your balance while maintaining your support with a chair.

Stand behind a chair with both hands on the head of the chair. Now place all your weight on one leg as you lift your other leg off the floor and out to the side. As you do this, shift your body weight onto the ball of your supporting leg, so you are on your tiptoes. Hold for 20 to 30 seconds, then release and change sides.

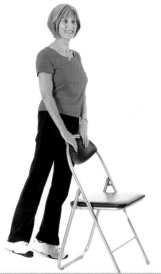

▶ **Variation**

To make the exercise more difficult you can take one hand off the chair. Or, to make it even more difficult, don't use a chair.

Seated Stability-Ball Balance

Level: Intermediate

Benefits: Improves your balance while also improving your seated posture.

Sit upright on a stability ball with your back straight and shoulders back and down. Place your feet about hip-width apart and, once stable, contract your abdominal muscles.

Exhale as you lift one foot off the floor and balance. You may need to stretch your arms out to your sides to help maintain balance. Breathe as you hold this position for 20 to 30 seconds, then swap legs and repeat.

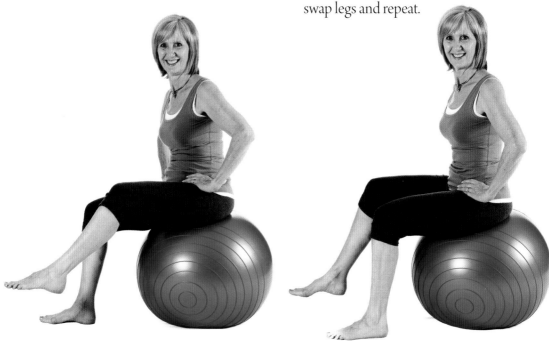

▶ **Tips**

Sitting up really tall and squeezing your abdominal muscles will help you with your balance.

If you find it difficult to get your balance, you can also rest a hand on the wall. Use the same hand as the leg you have raised off the floor.

Kneeling Stability-Ball Balance

Level: Advanced

Benefits: Improves your balance and core stability.

Start with a stability ball and chair in front of you. Gently guide the ball with your hands so you can place both knees about hip-width apart on the ball. Now roll your knees forward onto the ball so they are on top of the ball. As you do this, place your hand or hands on the chair to provide yourself with extra support. Try and keep your balance on the ball for 20 to 30 seconds. Then gently and slowly roll your knees off the ball.

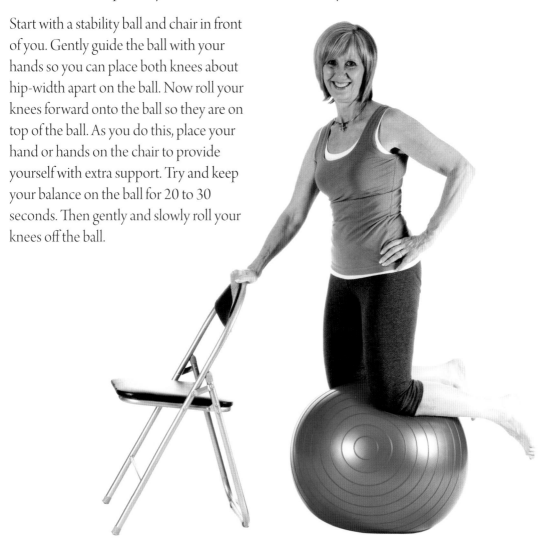

▶ **Variation**

To make the exercise harder you can take one hand or both hands off the chair to further increase the instability, and give your core muscles an even harder workout.

Tree Pose

Level: Intermediate to Advanced

Benefits: This is a challenging pose that will improve your strength and balance skills.

Stand tall in a neutral alignment. Your hips and shoulders should remain level throughout. Engage your core muscles by contracting your abdominals and lifting up your pelvic-floor muscles. Relax your shoulders down, and shift your body weight onto one foot. Then slowly bring the sole of your other foot up and rest it on the inner side of your other leg. It doesn't matter if you rest it above or below the knee; just do what feels more comfortable. Slowly bring your arms up straight to your sides, like a tightrope walker. Gently draw your bent-up knee out to the side. Look at a point ahead of you because this will help you maintain your focus and balance. Just relax and breathe as you maintain this pose for 20 to 30 seconds. Then return your foot back to the floor and your arms back down by your sides. Rest and then repeat the exercise using your other leg.

> ▶ **Tips**
>
> Ensure you pull your shoulders down when you do this exercise.
>
> You may want to look in a mirror to check out the levels of your shoulders and hips. If they are tilted, you can adjust them.

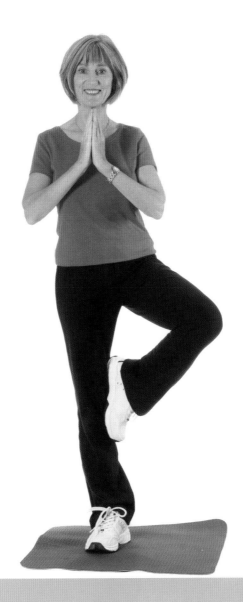

Once you feel comfortable and secure in your balance you can bring your hands together so that your palms are facing one another in front of your chest. This might challenge you, but it will improve your balance. Draw your shoulders down and shoulder blades together – this will lengthen your chest muscles.

If these exercises don't challenge you enough, you can make the pose more difficult by bringing your palms together above your head while still balancing on one leg.

Corner Balance

Benefits: Safely improves your sense of balance.

Stand in the corner of a room, with your back to the corner. Stand approximately 10 centimetres out from the wall, so if you do lose your balance, you won't fall too far. Place your feet so that one foot is further forward than the other – your front heel should be next to the toes of your back foot. Straighten your back and engage your core muscles. Look forward for about 10 breaths, focusing on a point in front of you. Next, cross your arms over in front of your chest. Hold this pose for 10 breaths, continuing to focus on a point ahead of you. Once you feel safe, try closing your eyes. You may feel a bit off-balance, but just concentrate on your breathing, relax and remember the walls aren't far away if needed. Repeat 3 times on each leg.

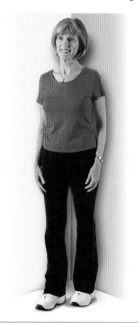 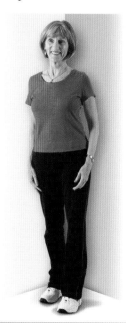 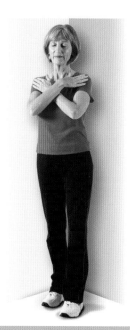

▶ **Tips**

You may be wobbly at first, but that's normal.

You'll find the more you practise, the more confident you will become, the stronger your feet, ankles and hip muscles will be, and the more your balance will evolve and improve.

Shifting the Weight from Foot to Foot

Benefits: An exercise that you use in your everyday life that strengthens your balance and weight-shifting skills.

Stand up with your shoulders back, and feet a bit wider than hip-width apart. Centre your upper body between your feet to start. Contract your abdominal muscles and take a few deep breaths to assist in gaining your concentration.

Slowly move your centre of gravity (which is about your belly button) to your right side, until it is directly above your right ankle. Your body weight should now be shifted onto the right foot. Keep your left foot on the ground to assist with maintaining your balance and ensure you keep your shoulders and hips level. Hold this pose for 20 to 30 seconds. Concentrate on contracting the muscles in your right leg and your gluteus medius muscles (located on the side of your hip).

Then move your weight back onto both feet. Rest, and repeat the exercise on your opposite leg.

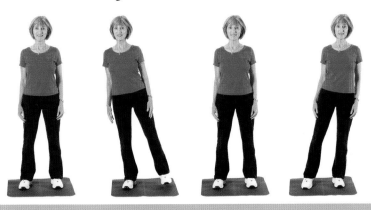

▶ **Tip**

Take your time, compose yourself and concentrate on the muscles contracting.

▶ **Variation**

Once you become increasingly confident with this exercise and your balance, challenge yourself to lifting your non-weight-bearing foot off the floor completely.

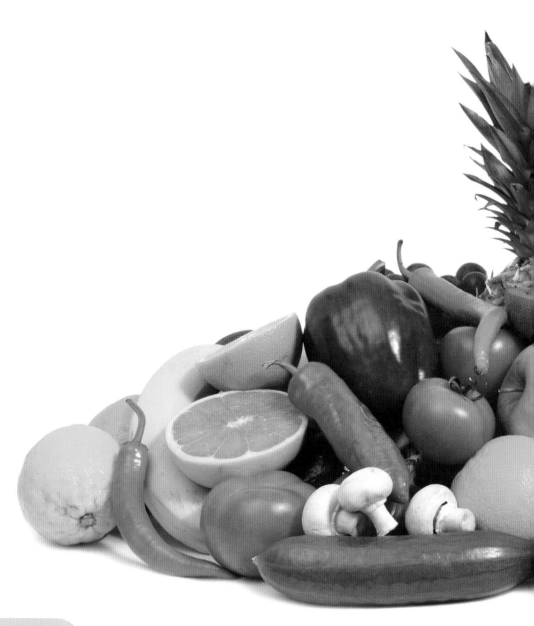

Chapter 12 Nutrition

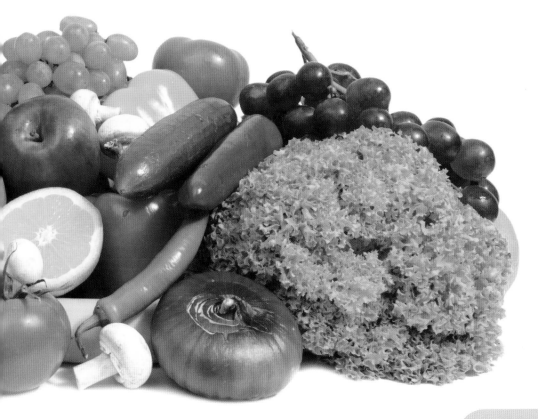

Introduction

Most of us are well aware of the importance of good nutrition, but with our hectic lifestyles, we often find ourselves too busy to take the time to select the right foods, and instead opt for less healthy, but more convenient options. Unfortunately these choices can have a detrimental impact on our overall health, wellbeing and ability to be productive.

Firstly, it is important that we hold ourselves accountable for the food choices that we make, and determine the reasons why we are consuming the particular foods we are. The question should be asked, why do I eat what I do? Am I eating for comfort, convenience or is it because I'm bored? Identify reasons and work on finding a solution to help you make the right choices in the future.

To help you along the way, it is essential to learn about what constitutes a healthy and nutritious diet. A healthy diet is outlined by the *Australian Guide to Healthy Eating*. This guide promotes sustainable healthy-eating habits that will assist you in reducing your risk of developing various health conditions such as type 2 diabetes, heart disease, certain cancers and other diseases and conditions. The guide is applicable to most individuals, but it will not necessarily suit individuals with certain health conditions. For further advice on dietary intake and for

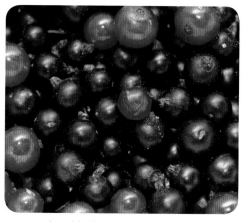

personalised help, it is advised you see a dietician.

The *Australian Guide to Healthy Eating* describes five food groups and recommends the types of foods and amounts of particular foods we should be eating on a daily basis. It also highlights the importance of eating a wide variety of healthy foods and drinking plenty of water. Furthermore, it recommends that you limit your intake of fatty food, salt and sugar. It is assumed that small portions of these will be eaten when consuming other food items such as breads and cereals. Hot chips, cakes, biscuits and sugary drinks should be limited to occasional consumption.

The five food groups identified by the *Australian Guide to Healthy Eating* are:

▶ Bread, cereals, rice, pasta, noodles

▶ Vegetables, legumes

▶ Fruit

▶ Milk, yoghurt, cheese

▶ Meat, fish, poultry, eggs, nuts, legumes

It is important to remember to balance your eating with your exercise. So when you are exercising, you may need extra food to help fuel your body so it can meet the extra demands being placed on it. It is a good idea to consult a dietician to give you advice on how much extra or less food you should be consuming in accordance to your exercise regime. Your overall goals of exercise will also impact on the types and amounts of food you should be consuming. For example, if you are overweight and trying to lose weight, you may need to reduce your kilojoule intake, and increase your level of physical activity.

Nutritional Tips

▶ Eat breakfast and don't skip meals.

▶ Reduce saturated-fat intake.

▶ Keep unhealthy foods such as cakes, hot chips and chocolate to a minimum.

▶ Eat lower-kilojoule foods such as whole grains, fruits and vegetables.

▶ Drink plenty of water.

▶ Eat smaller portions.

▶ Minimise added salt and foods high in salt.

▶ Limit your alcohol intake.

▶ Read food labels, especially for fat, sugar and kilojoule levels.

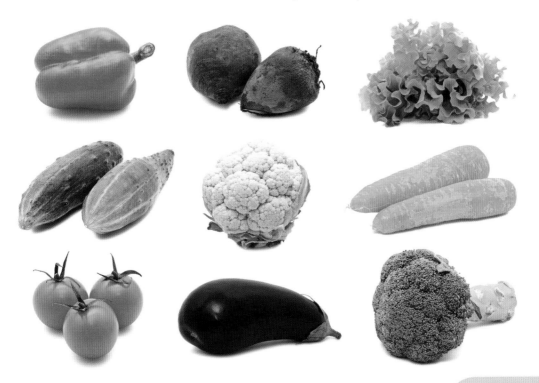

Recommended Daily Servings

	MEN		WOMEN	
	16 to 60 yrs	60 + yrs	16 to 60 yrs	60 + yrs
Cereals, breads, rice, pasta and noodles	6 to 12	4 to 9	4 to 9	4 to 7
Fruit	2	2	2	2
Vegetables and legumes	5	5	5	5
Milk, yoghurt and cheese	2	2	2	2
Lean meats, poultry, fish and alternatives	1	1	1	1
Extras (have no more than)	0 to 3	0 to 2.5	0 to 2.5	0 to 2

Serving Sizes

Cereals, breads, rice, pasta and noodles

- ▶ 2 slices of bread
- ▶ 1 cup of porridge
- ▶ 1 medium bread roll
- ▶ 1 cup of breakfast cereal
- ▶ 1 cup of cooked rice, pasta or noodles
- ▶ Half a cup of muesli

Fruit

- 1 piece of a medium-sized fruit, such as an apple, orange, banana, peach or pear
- 2 pieces of a smaller fruit such as kiwis, apricots, plums or figs
- Approximately 20 grapes or cherries
- Approximately 8 strawberries
- 1 cup of dried or canned fruit
- 1½ tablespoons of sultanas
- Half a cup of fruit juice
- Quarter of a medium melon or honeydew

Vegetables and legumes

- Half a cup of broccoli, cauliflower spinach, silverbeet, cabbage or sprouts
- 1 medium potato or half a medium sweet potato
- 1 cup of lettuce or salad vegetables
- Half a cup of beans, lentils or peas
- Half a cup of tomato, capsicum, cucumber, celery, eggplant, zucchini or mushroom
- 1 corn cob

Milk, yoghurt and cheese

- 250ml glass or a cup of milk (can be fresh, long-life or reconstituted)
- Half a cup of evaporated milk
- 1 cup of custard
- 2 slices of cheese
- A small tub of yoghurt (200g), plain or fruit

Meat, poultry, fish and alternatives

- 65–100g of cooked meat or chicken which is about a half a cup of mince, 2 small chops or 2 slices of roast meat
- 80–120g of cooked fish fillet
- 2 small eggs
- A third of a cup of canned beans, lentils, chickpeas, split peas or cooked beans
- A small handful of almonds or peanuts

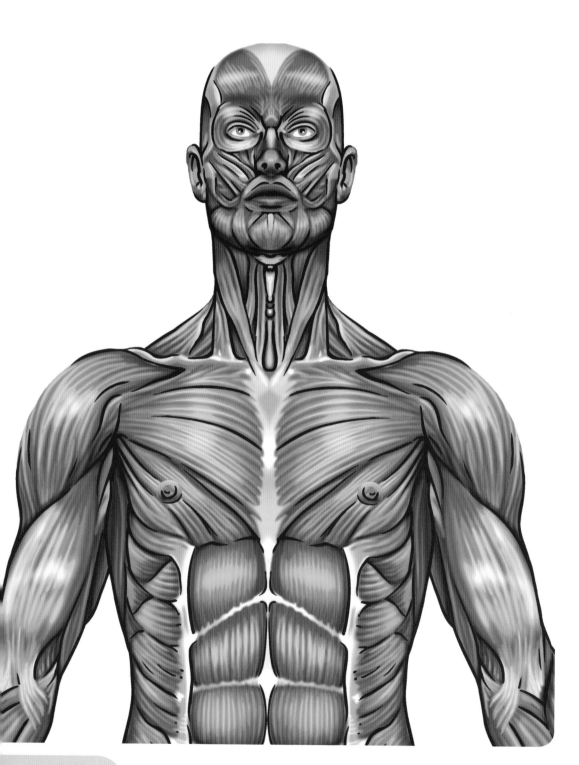

Chapter 13 Medical Conditions Associated with Nutrition and Exercise

Introduction

In this chapter we describe some of the medical conditions associated with age, inactivity and nutrition. Included is a description of sarcopenia, type 2 diabetes, osteoporosis, iron-deficiency anaemia and arthritis. Strength training can assist in reducing the risk of, or the progression of, some of these conditions. Discussed are ways to help minimise, prevent and manage these conditions.

Sarcopenia

Sarcopenia is the medical term used to describe age-related muscle loss, a very common occurrence. Throughout our adult life we lose muscles. This starts from about the age of 30, and on average we lose about 10 per cent of our lean muscle every 10 years. From the age of 60 this increases to 15 per cent every 10 years, then to 30 per cent every 10 years thereafter. The actual amount of muscle we lose will differ depending on our activity level and health.

This muscle loss leads to a reduction of our metabolic rate, which means that kilojoules that we were previously able to burn up by our muscles are stored as body fat, and this leads to weight gain.

This loss of muscle robs us of our functional health, independence and mobility, and further forces us into unhealthy and inactive lifestyles. This problem eventually pushes us into other lifestyle diseases such as high blood pressure, diabetes and heart disease.

This is a scary thought, but it is something we see, and are surrounded by, every day of our lives, whether in strangers, our loved ones or ourselves! But it doesn't have to be this way. Sarcopenia is reversible, and can be managed and minimised by exercise and strength training. Strength training is a proven way to increase muscle size and strength. So by increasing lean muscle you will speed up your metabolic rate, increasing your mobility and independence, which will lead to a longer, more independent and better-quality life.

Type 2 Diabetes

Type 2 diabetes is commonly described as a 'lifestyle disease' because it more commonly affects those who are overweight and inactive. It can also occur in those who have poor diets.

Type 2 diabetes occurs when the cells in your body don't respond to insulin (a sugar-lowering substance) properly, or the pancreas produces insufficient levels of insulin to meet the body's demands. When this happens, glucose (sugar) builds up in the blood stream, resulting in higher-than-normal blood-sugar levels.

Unfortunately, developing this disease can lead to multiple other health conditions and diseases. To reduce the risk of developing this disease it is important to eat healthy, reduce your sugar intake, participate in regular physical activity and maintain a healthy weight.

Osteoporosis

Osteoporosis is a disease of bone in which the bone mineral density is decreased. This unfortunately increases the risk of bone fractures and breaks. Osteoporosis is more prevalent in females, especially after menopause, but can also affect females and males of any age.

Once calcium is lost from the bones it is difficult to replace. However, changing your diet and increasing calcium, fluoride, vitamin D and strength training will assist in reducing your risk of developing the disease, or the progression of the condition. Calcium can be found in dairy products such as milk, cheeses and yoghurts. Furthermore, to help the absorption of calcium into your body, it is essential you get enough vitamin D. Thankfully vitamin D is free, and comes from the sun, so spending at least 20 minutes outside a day will help your body absorb calcium, and strengthen your bones.

Iron Deficiency Anaemia

Iron deficiency anaemia is a very common form of anaemia. It can affect people of any age and is caused by an insufficient dietary intake of iron, a loss of iron through bleeding or an increased demand for iron by the body. An iron deficiency leads to decreased haemoglobin production and subsequently impaired oxygen delivery within the body, because haemoglobin is what oxygen attaches itself to within the bloodstream. In some cases iron deficiency can be effectively managed by increasing the amount of iron in your diet. Foods that contain high levels of iron include red meats and green leafy vegetables.

Arthritis

Arthritis is a term used to describe more than 100 diseases, with the most common being osteoarthritis and rheumatoid arthritis. Arthritis is characterised by pain, swelling, heat, redness and reduced movement of a joint. It can affect anyone of any age.

Osteoarthritis arises when the cartilage that coats the ends of the bones, and acts as a shock absorber for the joints, breaks down. As this cartilage breaks down, the uncoated bones rub together, causing friction and resulting in pain.

Rheumatoid arthritis affects the lining of the joint's capsule known as the synovial tissue. This leads to deformities of the joint as the surrounding joint tissue becomes damaged. This condition can develop at any time, but predominantly occurs in the age group of 25 to 60 years.

Many people believe they shouldn't exercise when they have pain due to arthritis, thinking this will reduce their risk of further damage to their joints. In truth, no matter the severity of your arthritis, you should exercise regularly. Strength training is essential in reducing joint stress, as it helps with building up the muscles around the joint. Gentle, regular stretching is also crucial for the preservation of your range of movement.

On days when your joints are quite painful, take it easy, and ensure you take whatever anti-inflammatories your doctor has advised. These won't cure your problem, but they will make it easier for you to exercise and manage your condition. Alternatively, or in conjunction, you may like to use a heat pack to help with relieving your aches and improving your circulation.

At this time there is no cure for arthritis, but you can be proactive, protect your joints and reduce symptoms from worsening by keeping active and following a balanced workout plan.

Chapter 14 Posture and Lifting

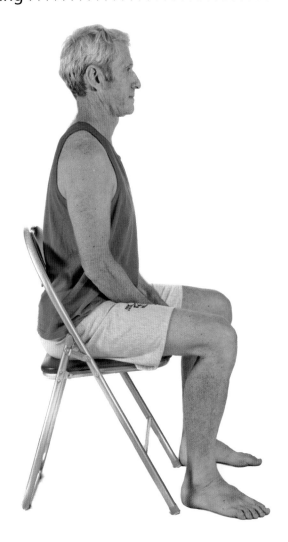

Introduction

Most people are aware that it is important to maintain good posture, and know what good posture is. However, at times we become complacent, ignoring our

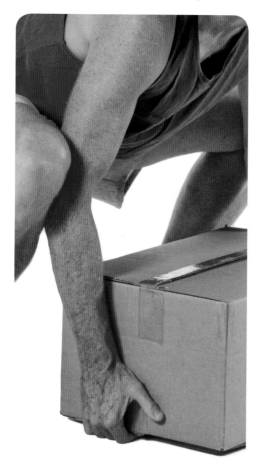

body's alignment, by slouching or lifting items incorrectly. When sitting and lifting it is important to concentrate on correct posture, as this will reduce your risk of sustaining an injury, and unnecessary muscle soreness and strain. This chapter provides examples of both bad and good posture, and outlines the proper ways to sit and lift.

Postural Alignment

When standing, it is important to remember not to slouch. The muscles are designed to lock the body in an upright position. This is when our body is at its strongest, as the muscles are supporting our bones and joints. When we slouch, there is much less support for the body, which can lead to long-term discomfort and back pain.

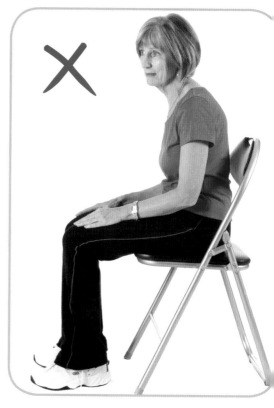

Sitting

Most of us, especially those who are seated for long periods of time, sit slumped with rolled shoulders and a curved back. As we all know how important it is to sit up straight, it is essential we keep reminding ourselves to correct our seated posture. When sitting, place your feet flat on the floor at hip-width apart, ensure your shoulders are square, and your back is straight.

Sitting on a stability ball may assist in strengthening your back muscles and improving your posture. As the ball is an unsteady object, thus causes you to use your stabilising muscles to maintain posture.

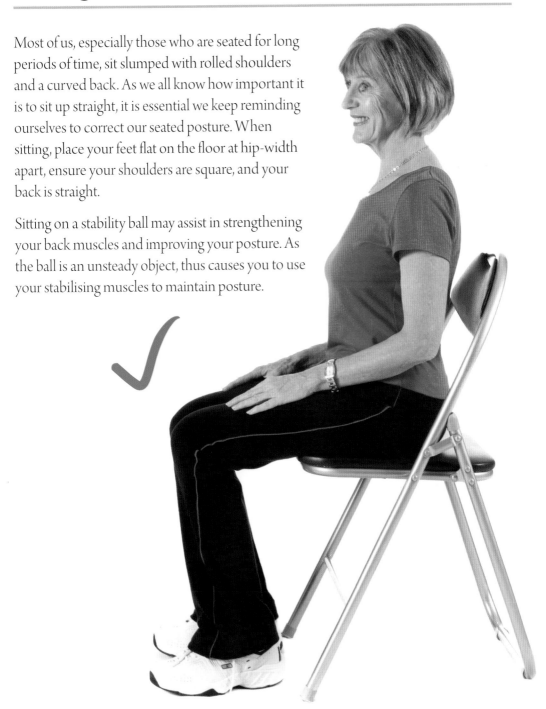

Lifting

Incorrect posture or technique when lifting an object is a common cause of back injury and can cause ongoing problems. The object you are lifting doesn't necessarily have to be heavy for back injuries to occur. When lifting, it is important to remember to use your legs to assist. Bend your knees while maintaining a straight back and keeping your chest up. Looking forward or up will help to keep your back straight. Grab hold of the object with your hands, then lift with your legs; ensure the weight goes through your heels and not your toes. This will help minimise the risk of any injury.

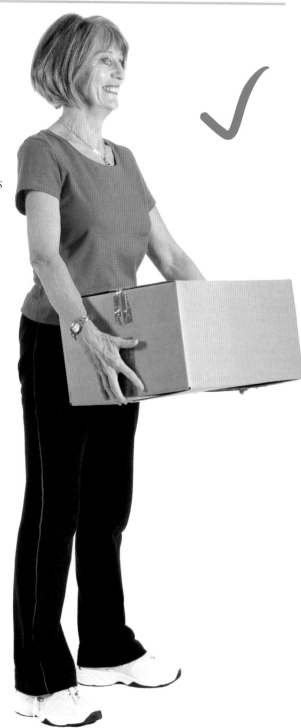

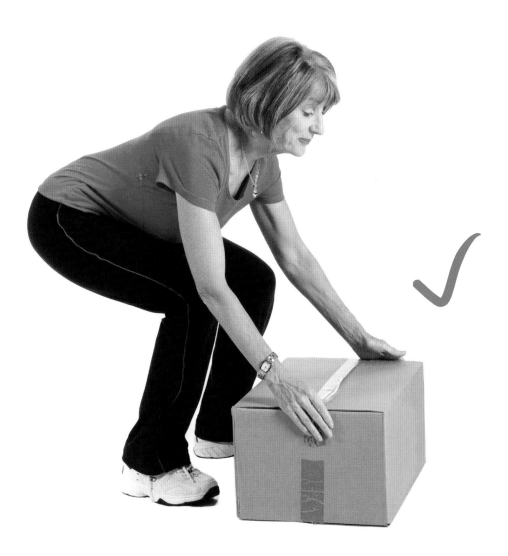

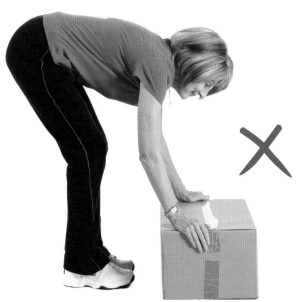

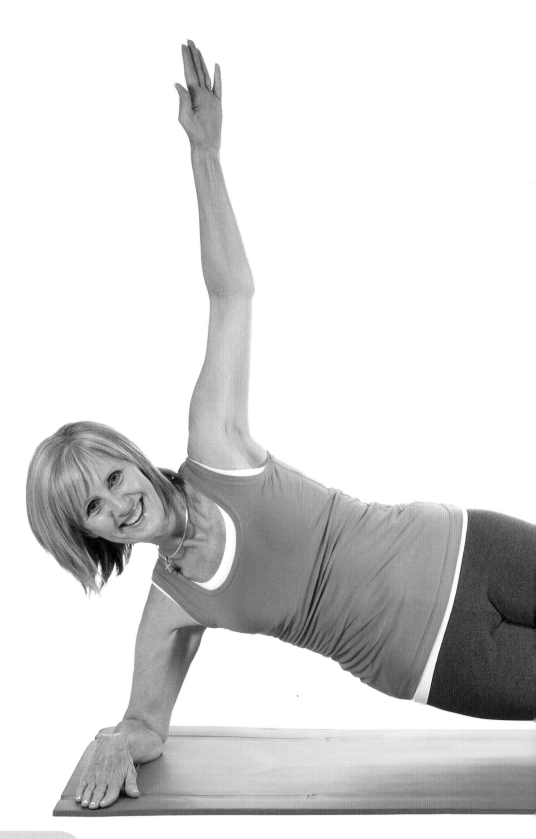

Chapter 15 Programs for All Levels

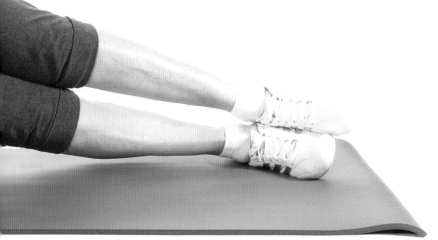

Cardio Program 1

Warm up for 10 to 15 minutes

See page 15 for warm-up exercises

Equipment

Step · Dumbbells · Mat

Exercise		Repetitions	Sets
Muscle Press	*See page 56*	15	3
Step-Up	*See page 33*	20	3
Push-Up on Toes	*See page 40*	15	3
Knee Lift	*See page 34*	15 each leg	3
Bent Row	*See page 48*	15	3
Jack Knife	*See page 83*	15	3
Step-Up	*See page 33*	20	3
The Plank	*See page 76*	30 seconds	3

Stretches

Hamstrings – Standing Hamstring Stretch · **Quadriceps** – Standing Quadricep Stretch · **Calves** – Standing Calf Stretch · **Back** – Leaning Stretch · **Shoulders** – Pull-Across Shoulder Stretch · **Chest** – Chest Wall Stretch · **Back** – Foetal Roll · **Back** – Child's Pose

Notes

Do each exercise one after the other with minimal or no rest in between. When you have completed all 8 exercises, rest for 1 minute, then repeat a further 2 times.

When stretching, hold each stretch for 20 to 30 seconds, and repeat each stretch twice.

Cardio Program 2

Warm up for 10 to 15 minutes
See page 15 for warm-up exercises

Equipment
Step · Dumbbells · Mat

Exercise	Repetitions	Sets
Single-Arm Lift *See page 58*	15	3
Knee to Elbows *See page 80*	20	3
Step-Up *See page 33*	60 seconds	3
Side Hover *See page 81*	30 secs each side	3
Knee Lift *See page 34*	15 each leg	3
Sit-Up *See page 78*	20	3
Bench Dip *See page 68*	15	3
Bicep Curl *See page 63*	15	3

Stretches

Chest – Chest Wall Stretch · **Back** – Back Stretch · **Shoulders** – Shoulder Two-Handed Stretch · **Bicep** – Bicep Stretch · **Tricep** – Tricep Stretch

Notes

Do each exercise one after the other with minimal or no rest in between. When you have completed all 8 exercises, rest for 1 minute, then repeat a further 2 times.
When stretching, hold each stretch for 20 to 30 seconds, and repeat each stretch twice.

Beginner Program for Upper Body

Warm up for 10 to 15 minutes

See page 15 for warm-up exercises

Equipment

Dumbbells · Mat · Chair

Exercise		Repetitions	Sets
Wall Push-Up	*See page 39*	12	3
Chair Row	*See page 49*	12	3
Shoulder Press	*See page 55*	12	3
Upright Row	*See page 57*	12	3
Bicep Curl	*See page 63*	12	3
Chair Dip	*See page 67*	12	3
Chair Leg Lift	*See page 71*	12	3
The Plank	*See page 76*	20 seconds	3

Stretches

Chest – Chest Wall Stretch · **Back** – Back Stretch · **Shoulders** – Shoulder Two-Handed Stretch · **Bicep** – Bicep Stretch · **Tricep** – Tricep Stretch

Notes

When performing the exercises you should do 2 in a row, then rest for 30 seconds. For example, do 12 wall push-ups followed by 12 chair rows, repeat this 3 times, and then move onto the next 2 exercises. When stretching, hold each stretch for 20 to 30 seconds, and repeat each stretch twice.

Beginner Program for Lower Body

Warm up for 10 to 15 minutes
See page 15 for warm-up exercises

Equipment
Ball · Chair · Mat · Step

Exercise		Repetitions	Sets
Ball Squat	*See page 26*	12	3
Leg Extension	*See page 29*	12	3
Floor Leg Curl	*See page 29*	12	3
Lying Leg Raise	*See page 31*	12	3
Pelvic Thrust	*See page 79*	12	3
Ball Crunch	*See page 72*	12	3
Step-Up	*See page 33*	30 seconds	3
The Plank	*See page 76*	20 seconds	3

Stretches
Hamstring – Floor Hamstring Stretch · **Quadriceps** – Lying Quadricep Stretch · **Groin** – Floor Groin Stretch · **Gluteal** – Gluteal Stretch · **Back** – Lying Twist

Notes
After each set have a 30-second rest. Complete all 3 sets before moving onto the next exercise. When stretching, hold each stretch for 20 to 30 seconds, and repeat each stretch twice.

Intermediate Program for Upper Body

Warm up for 10 to 15 minutes

See page 15 for warm-up exercises

Equipment

Dumbbells · Mat · Step

Exercise		Repetitions	Sets
Knee Push-Up	See page 41	12	3
One-Arm Row	See page 47	12	3
Muscle Press	See page 56	12	3
Upright Row	See page 57	12	3
Hammer Curl	See page 64	12	3
Kickback	See page 65	12	3
Bicycle Crunch	See page 82	12	3
Side Hover	See page 81	20 seconds	3

Stretches

Chest – Chest Wall Stretch · **Back** – Back Stretch · **Shoulders** – Shoulder Two-Handed Stretch · **Bicep** – Bicep Stretch · **Tricep** – Tricep Stretch

Notes

After each set have a 30-second rest. Complete all 3 sets before moving onto the next exercise. When stretching, hold each stretch for 20 to 30 seconds, and repeat each stretch twice.

Intermediate Program for Lower Body

Warm up for 10 to 15 minutes
See page 15 for warm-up exercises

Equipment
Chair · Dumbbell · Step · Mat

Exercise		Repetitions	Sets
Squat	*See page 25*	12	3
Sumo Squat	*See page 35*	12	3
Standing Leg Curl	*See page 28*	12	3
Leg Extension	*See page 29*	12	3
Knee Lift	*See page 34*	12	3
Ball Crunch	*See page 72*	12	3
Step-Up	*See page 33*	30 seconds	3
The Plank	*See page 76*	20 seconds	3

Stretches

Hamstring – Standing Hamstring Stretch · **Quadriceps** – Standing Quadricep Stretch · **Groin** – Standing Groin Stretch · **Gluteal** – Gluteal Stretch · **Back** – Lying Twist

Notes

After each set have a 30-second rest. Complete all 3 sets before moving onto the next exercise. When stretching, hold each stretch for 20 to 30 seconds, and repeat each stretch twice.

Advanced Program for Upper Body

Warm up for 10 to 15 minutes
See page 15 for warm-up exercises

Equipment
Dumbbells · Mat · Chair

Exercise	Repetitions	Sets
Push-Up on Toes *See page 40*	12	4
Chest Fly *See page 43*	12	4
Bent Row *See page 48*	12	4
The Wood Chopper *See page 51*	12	4
Shoulder Press *See page 55*	12	4
Reverse Fly *See page 50*	12	4
Hammer Curl *See page 64*	12	4
Tricep Extension *See page 66*	12	4

Stretches

Chest – Chest Wall Stretch · **Back** – Back Stretch · **Shoulders** – Pull-Across Shoulder Stretch
· **Bicep** – Bicep Stretch · **Tricep** – Tricep Stretch

Notes

When performing the exercises you should do 2 in a row, then rest for 30 seconds. For example, do 12 push-ups on toes followed by 12 chest flies. Repeat this 4 times, and then move onto the next 2 exercises. When stretching, hold each stretch for 20 to 30 seconds, and repeat each stretch twice.

Advanced Program for Lower Body

Warm up for 10 to 15 minutes

See page 15 for warm-up exercises

Equipment

Mat · Chair · Ball · Step

Exercise		Repetitions	Sets
Squat	*See page 25*	12	4
One-Leg Ball Squat	*See page 27*	12	4
Lunge	*See page 32*	12	4
Standing Leg Raise	*See page 30*	12	4
Knee Lift	*See page 34*	12	4
Knee to Elbows	*See page 80*	12	3
Jack Knife	*See page 83*	12	3
The Plank	*See page 76*	20 seconds	3

Stretches

Hamstring – Standing Hamstring Stretch · **Quadriceps** – Standing Quadricep Stretch · **Groin** – Standing Groin Stretch · **Gluteal** – Gluteal Stretch · **Back** – Lying Twist

Notes

After each set have a 30-second rest. Complete all 4 sets before moving onto the next exercise. When stretching, hold each stretch for 20 to 30 seconds, and repeat each stretch twice.

Quick Full-Body Program

Warm up for 10 to 15 minutes
See page 15 for warm-up exercises

Equipment
Chair · Dumbbells · Mat

Exercise	Repetitions	Sets
Chair Row *See page 49*	15	3
Leg Extension *See page 29*	15	3
Shoulder Press *See page 55*	15	3
Squat *See page 25*	15	3
Chair Dip *See page 67*	15	3
Standing Leg Curl *See page 28*	15	3
Standing Leg Raise *See page 30*	15	3
Chair Balance *See page 115*	30 seconds	3

Stretches

Back – Leaning Stretch · **Hamstrings** – Seated Hamstring Stretch · **Quadriceps** – Assisted Quadricep Stretch · **Shoulder** – Shoulder Two-Handed Stretch · **Tricep** – Tricep Stretch · **Back** – Downward FacingDog

Notes

When performing the exercises you should do 2 in a row, then rest for 30 seconds. For example, do 15 chair rows followed by 15 leg extensions. Repeat this 3 times, and then move onto the next 2 exercises. When stretching, hold each stretch for 20 to 30 seconds, and repeat each stretch twice.

Abdominal Program

Warm up for 10 to 15 minutes
See page 15 for warm-up exercises

Equipment
Mat · Ball

Exercise	Repetitions	Sets
Ball Crunch See page 72	12	3
Ball Twist See page 73	12	3
Pelvic Thrust See page 79	12	3
Back Stabilising or Bird Dog See page 74	20 seconds	3
Side Hover See page 81	20 seconds	3

Stretches
Child's Pose · Foetal Roll · Lying Twist · Downward Facing Dog

Notes
After each set have a 30-second rest. Complete all 3 sets before moving onto the next exercise. When stretching, hold each stretch for 20 to 30 seconds, and repeat each stretch twice.

Beginner Balance Program

Warm up for 10 to 15 minutes

See page 15 for warm-up exercises

Equipment

Mat • Chair

Exercise	Repetitions	Sets
Shifting the Weight from Foot to Foot *See page 121*	20 seconds	3
Chair Balance *See page 115*	20 seconds	3
Tree Pose *See page 118*	20 seconds	3
Back Stabilising or Bird Dog *See page 74*	20 seconds	3
Side Hover *See page 81*	20 seconds	3

Stretches

Child's Pose • Foetal Roll • Lying Twist • Downward Facing Dog

Notes

After each set have a 30-second rest. Complete all 3 sets before moving onto the next exercise. When stretching, hold each stretch for 20 to 30 seconds, and repeat each stretch twice.

Advanced Balance Program

Warm up for 10 to 15 minutes
See page 15 for warm-up exercises

Equipment
Mat · Chair · Ball

Exercise		Repetitions	Sets
Tree Pose	See page 118	30 seconds	3
Seated Stability-Ball Balance	See page 116	30 seconds	3
Kneeling Stability-Ball Balance	See page 117	30 seconds	3
Back Stabilising or Bird Dog	See page 74	30 seconds	3
Side Hover	See page 81	30 seconds	3

Stretches
Child's Pose · Foetal Roll · Lying Twist · Downward Facing Dog

Notes
After each set have a 30-second rest. Complete all 3 sets before moving onto the next exercise. When stretching, hold each stretch for 20 to 30 seconds, and repeat each stretch twice.

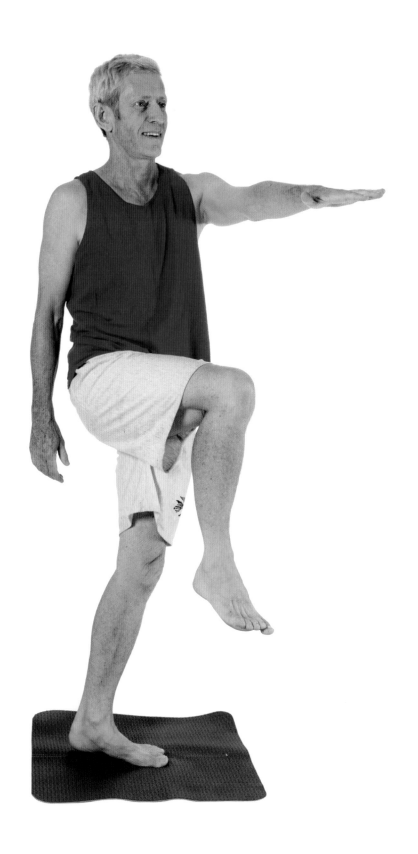

Chapter 16 Muscle Soreness and Alternative Forms of Exercise

Muscle Soreness

Muscle soreness often occurs after vigorous activity, normally the following day. This is called 'delayed onset of muscle soreness' (DOMS). The extent of your DOMS will depend on your activity type, and the intensity and duration of the activity. The harder and heavier you work, the greater the DOMS.

There are three main contractions or actions your muscles make: concentric, eccentric and isometric.

▶ Concentric is the shortening of the muscle when it is contracting.

▶ Eccentric is the lengthening of the muscle when it is contracting.

▶ Isometric is when the muscle contracts while there is no movement.

For example, when squatting, on the way down would be an eccentric contraction, while holding the squat at the bottom of the movement would be an isometric contraction, and on the way back up would be a concentric contraction.

DOMS normally occurs with slow, controlled eccentric movements – the eccentric phase is when most of the muscle damage occurs.

Ways to Reduce Muscle Soreness

Doing an appropriate warm-up will reduce the chances of severe DOMS. This normally consists of low- to medium-intensity exercise for 10 to 20 minutes. If you are a beginner, it is suggested you warm up for at least 20 minutes prior to commencing your

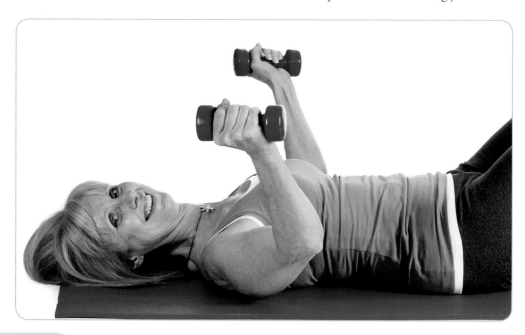

exercise regime because you are more likely to be subject to DOMS.

Increase weight by small increments of about 0.5 kilogram to 1 kilogram at a time. Allow sufficient recovery between sessions. Stretch and cool down appropriately.

Cooling down is just as important as the exercise itself. This should consist of a full range of movement at a low intensity, such as walking and then stretching the body parts that you have worked. Stretches should be held for 15 to 30 seconds, and repeated 2 to 3 times each.

Nutrition also plays a massive role in reducing DOMS because when you exercise you deplete your stored glucose (sugar) levels. An average person has approximately 60 grams of stored sugar in their body, which takes about 20 minutes to deplete. Studies have shown that replacing these sugar levels dramatically increases your recovery rate, therefore reducing your chances of DOMS.

You also need to replace protein after exercise. Protein is very important for muscle recovery. Our body does not store protein so it is important to have small serves throughout the day. As we exercise, amino acids (proteins) escape from muscle cells as they are damaged so we need to replace these proteins for the cells to be able to recover. A protein-rich meal, shake or smoothie (preferably a liquid-based protein because it is absorbed quickly) within one hour of exercise should be consumed, and this will dramatically decrease your chances of soreness.

Alternative Forms of Exercise

Have you ever thought about taking part in an alternative form of exercise? These are just a few other ways you can reach your goals and maintain your motivation.

Tai Chi

Tai chi is a Chinese martial art which was developed at least 300 years ago, but may have originated about 2000 years ago. It has been described as the physical expression of the spirit and principles of Taoism. It is a set of exercises, or specific carefully orchestrated movements, that take on the appearance of an array of dances. It is often practised in groups, with everyone performing precisely the same movements at the same time.

Unlike other forms of martial arts, including judo and karate, tai chi is a non-contact, non-combative way of improving health and energy, and reducing stress. Its practice promotes flexibility, balance and physical control.

Tai chi is also a kind of moving meditation, where the mind centres itself on each movement, producing inner calm. The tai chi exercises improve the energy flow (chi) within the body.

Yoga

Yoga is an ancient system of breathing practices, physical exercises, postures and meditation intended to integrate the individual's body, mind and spirit. It originated in India several thousand years ago, and its principles were first written down by a scholar named Patanjali in the second century BC. The word yoga comes from a Sanskrit word, *yukti*, and means 'union' or 'yoke'.

Yoga is an integration of the mental, physical and spiritual dimensions of life. The stretching, bending and balancing involved in the physical postures of yoga help to align the head and spinal column; stimulate the circulatory system, endocrine glands and other organs; and keep muscles and joints strong and flexible. Yoga programs have been shown to reduce the risk of heart disease by lowering blood pressure and anxiety levels.

Pilates

Pilates is a body-conditioning technique designed to stretch, strengthen and balance the body. It targets the deep postural muscles within the body through a series of exercises aimed at building muscle strength and rebalancing the body. It is excellent for improving posture, core strength and flexibility and for aligning the body correctly. Pilates also teaches co-ordination, concentration and control of the body.

About the Author

John Forde grew up in country Victoria, one of nine children. He always had a passion for fitness and being social, whether it was playing footy with his mates, lifting weights with his dad or proving he was the strongest of his siblings. John went on to study gym instruction and personal training, including undertaking specialities in training children and older adults. He has worked in aged care and community health, and now lectures in fitness, as well as running a health-and-fitness store.

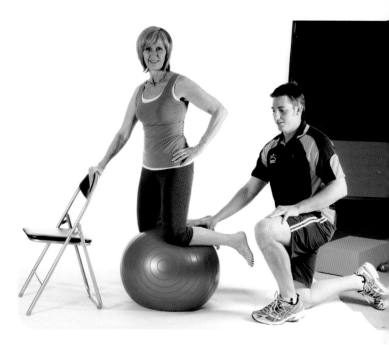

Acknowledgements

Special thanks go to my wife Laura, my direct family and in-laws, my peers and my students who have supported me over the years by keeping me motivated and inspired throughout my training, further studies, teaching and the starting of my own business.

Teaching people about fitness and its benefits is a very fulfilling profession, and I hope to share this passion with you, and inspire you to be proactive in improving your health and the health of your family and friends.

About the Photographer

Peter Bourne is a graphic designer/photographer who specialises in editorial photography. The photographs in this book were taken in the offices of the publisher (The Five Mile Press) using an Elinchrom BX500 portable lighting system and processed with Adobe Lightroom. He lives overlooking Melbourne in the Dandenong Ranges, east of the city.

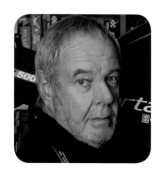

Nikon D300; Nikkor 17–55 AF-S DX; f/2.8

Index

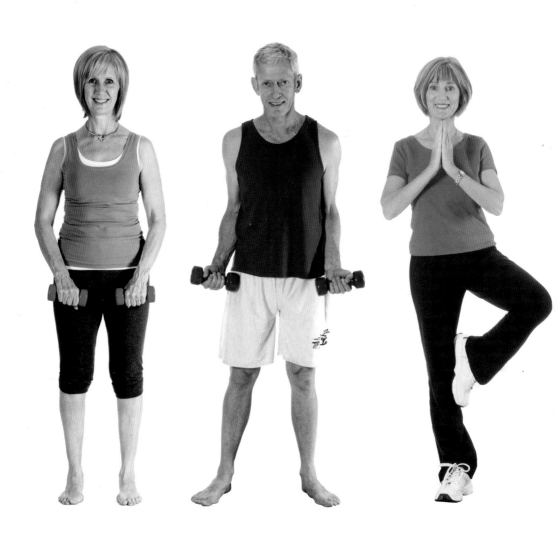